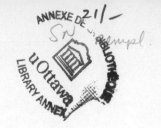

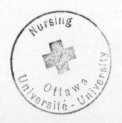

TOPICS IN PUBLIC HEALTH

A

TOPICS IN
PUBLIC HEALTH

by

J. M. MACKINTOSH
M.D., D.P.H.

E. & S. LIVINGSTONE LTD.
EDINBURGH AND LONDON
1965

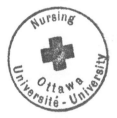

RA
425
· M32
1965

ACKNOWLEDGMENTS

I wish to thank The Avalon Foundation and the Milbank Memorial Fund for their assistance and especially for the encouragement which I received from Dr. Thomas Parran and Dr. Frank G. Boudreau who were at that time the Presidents of those two Foundations.

I also have pleasure in acknowledging the great help which I have received at various times from Helen Papworth, Betty Vorwald and Joan Lynes, who were of immense assistance, especially when the shadows began to fall.

The greater part of the essays were written for the American Hospital Association and I am grateful for their help in publishing.

1965.   *J. M. M.*

CONTENTS

Chapter		Page
I	The Roots of Progress	1
II	Hospital Care	12
III	The State and The Child	29
IV	Social Diagnosis	52
V	Teaching and Practice of Public Health	59
VI	The Physically Handicapped	76
VII	Mental Health in Public Health Practice	94
VIII	Housing	112
IX	Voluntary Service	130
X	Medicine as a Social Science	142
XI	Health Education	152
XII	Care of the Aged	158
XIII	Accidents as a World Problem	175
XIV	Damage in the New Towns	189
XV	The Meaning and Scope of a Public Health Service	241
XVI	Medical Care Tomorrow	254
XVII	Out of the Shadows	266
XVIII	The Swing of the Pendulum	273
XIX	American Pilgrimage in Wartime	279

Chapter 1

THE ROOTS OF PROGRESS

It has been customary in dealing with the history of public health to distinguish rather sharply between two periods: The age of environmental progress, which in England occupied approximately the second half of the nineteenth century, and the age of personal health, which corresponds roughly with the first half of the twentieth. It is generally admitted that the eighteenth century was a period of individualism, starred with pioneer work in prevention; and that the first half of the nineteenth century was a time of trial and confusion following the industrial revolution. During this period factors inducing ill-health, such as bad housing and insanitary factories, were gradually eliminated in preparation for the advances of the environmental age. In reviewing the later half of the nineteenth century, Sir John Simon was able to strike a cheerful note in reference to the advance of law and order, and especially as regards public education in health standards and practices. He praised above all a growing self-helpfulness of the 'proletariat' and their enlarging sense of 'socialistic' duty; that is, the constantly increasing care for the community at large. This is in sharp contrast with the conditions of the first half of the century, which represented a large area of misery and regression which was associated with the worst features of the industrial revolution in England. For an estimate of this earlier period the assessment of J. L. and Barbara Hammond is harsh, but true:—

Amid the great distress that followed Waterloo and peace, it was a commonplace of men like Castlereagh and Canning that England was the only happy country in the world, and that so long as the monopoly of their little class was left untouched, her happiness would survive. That class has left bright and ample records of its life in literature, in art, in political traditions, in the display of great orations and debates, in memories of brilliant conversation and sparkling wit; it has left dim and meagre records of the disinherited peasants that are the shadow of its wealth; of the exiled labourers that are the shadow of its pleasures; of the villages sinking in poverty and crime and shame that are the shadow of its power and its pride.[1]

There is perhaps some confusion in the fact that England is so often chosen as representing the rise of industrial health. It is not that this country was specially advanced in this respect at the beginning of the period, but rather the reverse. England was one of the first countries to make the change from a predominantly agricultural to an industrial economy. This great movement, commonly called the industrial revolution, unhappily swept over a land entirely unprepared for the event; neither central nor local government was ready to cope with these vast changes, and the prevailing economic theories were weighted against sanitary legislation. The battle for public health could hardly have begun at a more inauspicious time, but, as Sydney Smith pointed out, this is the common situation:

> Which is the properest day to do good? Which is the properest day to remove a nuisance? We answer, the very first day a man can be found to propose the removal of it; and whoever opposes the removal of it on that day will (if he dare) oppose it on every other. There is in the minds of many feeble friends to virtue and improvement an imaginary period for the removal of evils, which it would certainly be worth while to wait for, if there was the smallest chance of its ever arriving—a period of unexampled peace and prosperity when a patriotic king and an enlightened mob united their ardent efforts for the amelioration of human affairs; when the oppressor is as delighted to give up the oppression as the oppressed is to be liberated from it; when the difficulty and the unpopularity would be to continue the evil, not to abolish it! These are the periods when fair-weather philosophers are willing to venture out and hazard a little for the general good. But the history of human nature is so contrary to all this, that almost all improvements are made after the bitterest resistance, and in the midst of tumults and civil violence—the worst period at which they can be made, compared to which any period is eligible and should be seized hold of by the friends of salutary reform.[2]

The industrial revolution was well under way before the end of the eighteenth century, but the battle for public health did not even begin until 1838, after much of the environmental damage had been done. The contribution of Simon's thought and action towards the alleviation of poverty in the developing industrial towns can hardly be over-estimated. In dealing with the politics of poverty, he drew special attention throughout his career to the lives of the poorest workers and the privations which they had to endure. In this own rather humble commentary he points out that in the years 1864-66 he submitted for presentation to Parliament

> masses of evidence, both rural and urban, often of the most painful character, as to the very meagre nourishment on which low-priced labour is done, and as to the frequent extreme want of proper housing for local quantities of labouring population.[3]

In this respect Chadwick, Simon and their colleagues had a clear concept of the triple relationship of poverty, ill-health and bad housing, and an appreciation of the fact that children were the main cause of poverty. It is pathetic to see that in the developing world of today just the same errors of omission and commission are being made—the mad rush to set up a town where treasures of the earth have been discovered or a water supply developed, without any preparation for the health and comfort of the employees, and without even the elements of protective legislation.

Again and again in the history as it unfolds of the development of a new country, one finds the same unhappy sequence of events. First of all there is the clamour for independence, followed by the rush for power. The next event to rear its head is the rise of industry and the scandalous failure of authority to meet the inevitable conflict of the interests of the landowners, jerry builders, and contractors for public services.

People who look back into history from the vantage point of today are apt to think that England in the first half of the nineteenth century was a poor little country, struggling against poverty and unable to afford any great expenditure on public health. The reverse is the case. As represented by the Great Exhibition of 1851, England was at the height of her prosperity. All the world came to admire her wealth, progress and enlightenment—that thrice happy realm which had escaped the continental revolutions of 1848. It was in that year that 'The Economist' wrote, in opposing the Public Health Act:

> Suffering and evil are nature's admonitions. They cannot be

got rid of; and the impatient attempts of benevolence to banish them from the world by legislation before benevolence has learnt their object and their end, have always been more productive of evil than good.

It is of melancholy significance to observe that during that period, when few towns had a water supply, or sewers, or paved or lighted streets, or homes worth the name, Railway Construction Bills went through Parliament to the tune of three hundred million pounds. The amount borrowed for public health in the same period was less than three million pounds. The situation has changed today in favour of road works, but the lesson is the same.

No doubt the widespread misery and destitution of this period in England and in other advancing countries were due to multiple causes: the sudden transition from domestic to factory employment; the uncontrolled influx of workers and of those seeking work to the new towns; houses constructed without the shadow of control by public authorities. These causes, however, are apt to repeat themselves time and again in different countries, and the denial of health to the people is the product of a laissez faire individualism which allows almost unlimited scope for the exploitation of the weak. Unfortunately such factors which are prominent in many of the new countries today are relatively neglected.

England's prosperity reached its height about 1870, but after that a number of influences led to a decline in relation to industrial development, and more particularly foreign trade. This was eclipsed to some extent by the general rise in wage level and the growth in prosperity in the new middle classes. During the last quarter of the century, however, increasing competition from abroad, especially by the imposition of tariffs, steadily undermined the position of foreign trade for Britain. The check to national productivity towards the end of the century has been ably explained by Marshall, the economist, and recorded by Ensor in his book 'England 1870-1914', as due to the loss of industrial leadership and the failure of the country to adapt its industrial machines to the new conditions in Europe and the colonies. This was the outward and visible change, but within the country itself there were more serious hindrances to the forward movement. The most striking of these, as we have seen, was the poor physical condition of the workers and their children and the wretched and overcrowded housing conditions.

In the world today we are facing the wider challenge of industrial health. I use the word 'challenge' to make it clear that I am discussing only a very limited section of a vast subject. What is meant here is the challenge that industrial health offers to public health practice—to be ignored only at peril to the community. It could indeed be said that the rise of public health in the nineteenth century would have afforded comparatively few problems to the public authorities if there had not been an industrial revolution. This can be seen at once by comparative studies of countries in which industrial changes have only just begun to take place—and how sadly unready they are to meet them. The only comfort is that their situation would have been far worse but for the watchfulness and help of international bodies such as the International Labour Office and the World Health Organization.

Industrial revolutions have been enemies of health, when they might have been close friends through careful organization in advance. No doubt this was to be wise after the event, but in this case the event has taken place again and again through nearly two centuries without the early introduction of preventive measures. The worst features of the case are that no advance preparation is made by any educational means among health authorities or through any of the usual educational channels in schools or elsewhere. To take a recent example: during housing developments between the wars, some of the more advanced authorities took the step of demonstrating the various types of homes to prospective tenants, and in this way ignorant destruction was avoided. Soon after the tenants had been installed, skilled housing managers visited them and solved many of their problems of care and management. But a vast number of authorities throughout the world could not have cared less. They paid no real attention to their guests, with the result that they reaped in both town and country a sodden harvest of dirt, damage and disorder.

Today in many parts of Europe there is a fair degree of control over the conditions of the larger industrial developments; but in the smaller factories, which sometimes reach ninety per cent of the total, there is little advance and practically no inspection.

Public health and industrial health cannot be separated on any logical principle. It is therefore essential to have the closest possible liaison between the general health officer and his colleague in industry. There problems differ sharply, however, because the industrial health officer requires highly specialised training to meet the needs of medicine in modern industry, while the health officer is concerned primarily with the general community.

There is a further problem in the rising countries of today. The replacement of small by large scale enterprise has altered the physical conditions of work from the dominance of the individual to the membership of the group. Perhaps the most striking feature from the health point of view is the continuous rise in the total production of goods, leading to a demand far beyond the factories of a single country. This has of course attracted to the industrial areas millions of immigrants who have to be absorbed in housing and in industrial relationships, as well as personal habits. The admission of aliens has greatly complicated the task of absorption, and the labourer is in general more and more separated from his source of food supply and is dependent directly on money wages. In this respect, social organization has become incomparably more important and is making human sympathy a power in politics. In the earlier days public health authorities felt that it was their main duty to offer a definite though limited place for private benevolence so long as it was organized in such a way as to discourage thriftlessness and laziness. In the world of today voluntary movements have a position of great importance, but it is more associated with service than with contributions in money. In other words, the Governments of many countries, whatever their political adherence may be, have to offer greater support, by way of insurance or at least provision against poverty, injury, old age, as well as providing against unemployment.

To return to the nineteenth century for a moment, the third quarter served a valuable function in two main respects: the promotion of scientific investigation and the rapid spread of knowledge gained by skilled enquiry and research through the more advanced countries in the world. Until recently, less attention has been given to the influence of that period in administrative and social advances under the leadership of men like Simon in England, Pettenkofer in Germany and Shattuck in the United States. This extension of health practice found its way to the far corners of the earth through constantly increasing contacts of human beings, and in this respect colonial development made very remarkable contributions to sanitation, cleansing, water supplies and housing and laid the foundations for the personal health services of the twentieth century. In one respect, however, the sanitary reformers of the previous century, who contributed mainly to the public health legislation of that time, tended to believe that improved sanitation alone would bring down the death rates and the infant mortality in a very short time. In this they were disappointed, as there was little change in the decades which immediately followed the public health Acts. As it turned out, other factors associated with ill health had been relatively neglected: bad housing, overcrowding, poor nutrition and long hours of work, and the delay in securing skilled care for mothers and children.

The twentieth century has been rightly described as the age of 'personal and community health'. Sidney Webb, the economist, writing in 1901, said enthusiastically 'This time it is *not* a new continent that the ordinary man has discovered, but a new *category*. We have become aware almost in a flash that we are not merely individuals, but members of a community, nay, citizens of the world. . . . In short, the opening of the twentieth century finds us all, to the dismay of the old-fashioned individualist, thinking in communities.'

Sidney Webb was too optimistic as regards time, because he was in a hurry, but he was unerring in seeing the trend of social development. Two events had stimulated new thinking. First, a series of social investigations of a scientific kind, notably the work of Charles Booth on the Population of London, and the more accurate but limited study by Rowntree on the City of York. The second event was a sharp increase of public anxiety about the physical health of the people. In the year 1902, General Sir Frederick Maurice wrote an article entitled 'Where to Get Men', and he said that out of every five men wishing to enlist for service in the South African War, only two remained effective soldiers after two years. These disclosures stirred the

Government to appoint an Interdepartmental Committee in the year 1903. Modern personal hygiene begins with the recommendations of this Committee, whose advice deserves close study. The findings are not confident, largely for lack of material on which to base judgments. In general the Committee reported that the physical condition of the poorer classes in the towns was very bad, but capable of rapid improvement:

> Laziness, want of thrift, ignorance of household management, and in particular the choice and preparation of food; filth, indifference to parental obligations, and drunkenness largely infect adults of both sexes, and press with terrible severity on their children.

They condemned in plain terms the manner and the spirit in which the Local Government Board did its health work.

'The public health is a matter of the highest general concern', they say, and go on to express a firm belief in the soundness of the principle of delegation of health functions to local authorities; but they hold no less strongly that an important function remains for the Central Government as representing the nation at large, viz:

> to watch the play of local administration throughout the country and to bring influence to bear on backward districts, with a view to levelling them up to the standards attained in what are by general consent the best administered areas. They venture to doubt whether this latter consideration had received due prominence. The mass of routine work in which the Local Government Board is immersed affords it little time for the consideration of questions of public policy in the sphere of health, and may render it slow to assume the responsibility of applying new principles of administration; but it is in these directions that opportunities for improvement lie. . .

> The Committee are given to understand that the pressure from above, which in many cases they consider so necessary, is very intermittently employed; indeed, in some spheres of the Board's possible activity, the powers conferred are held in permanent suspense. Thus in no case, with a view to compelling the enforcement by the local authority of any provisions of the Act which it is their duty to enforce, has the Board ever made an order under S.229 of the Public Health Act, 1875, limiting the time for the performance of their duty by the local authority; nor has an order ever been issued under S.31 of the Housing Act, 1890, Part II, even if, as seems doubtful, any such order is enforceable.

In other words, the Local Government Board had been grossly neglecting its public health duties. In London, for example, the low standard of 300 cubic feet of space for adults in bedrooms was not enforced, and in most towns innumerable sanitary provisions of the most elementary kind were neglected without any protest from the Local Government Board.

The Committee went on to make a series of remarkable recommendations, some of which have not even yet been put into effect:

1. *A register of sickness,* not confined to communicable disease. This valuable recommendation has not yet been carried out.

2. *Overcrowding.* The Committee said that the time had come to deal drastically with overcrowding and urged that local authorities should establish minimum standards and see that they were enforced. This measure reached the Statute Book in 1935.

3. *Infant Mortality.* The Committee said that the connection between overcrowding and bad or insufficient feeding had been established. They strongly recommended an improvement in the statistics of infant life and death, including the registration of stillbirths. This was actually recommended by the Brussels Conference on Hygiene in 1903, but it was not established as a legal requirement in Great Britain until a quarter of a century later.

4. *Better Training of Mothers.* The Committee recommended that, as models for maintaining and improving on this step already existed, it required only careful study and a genuine faith in the value of social education to bring this training into general use.

In Britain, it took a matter of twenty years to get this recommendation accepted. The Committee laid a good deal of stress upon the value of public health nurses, especially in home visitation and in the teaching of mothers. A startling suggestion was that the schools should be used for giving lessons in motherhood to girls. I doubt if this has been accepted even now, except as a local effort.

5. *Mothers at work.* The Committee were divided about the risks involved in mothers of young children going out to work; but the majority felt that, if the local authorities established day-nurseries for the benefit of mothers at work, any risk would be greatly diminished. In England, these day nurseries have been widely established since the second World War and have been wholly beneficial. The fear that they might help to spread

infectious disease among young children has not in fact been realized.

6. *School leaving age.* The Committee strongly recommended an extension of the school leaving age for the purpose of instructing older girls in cookery, domestic work and home hygiene, and they insisted that properly qualified teachers should be used for the purpose. This useful recommendation was slowly introduced into the English schools but it seems to me a pity that they did not advise that boys also should be trained in domestic jobs, especially in minor household repairs and general help in the home.

7. *Medical Inspection of School Children.* The Committee recommended general medical inspection of school children with particular reference to care of the teeth, eyes and ears. This recommendation was the first to be put into action—about four years afterwards.

8. *Protection of Food.* A great deal of attention was given to standards of feeding and the Committee recommended official standards of purity for foods and drinks. They spoke especially about the dangers of foul milk, both in the dairy and at home.

9. *Industrial Health Services.* Finally, the Committee pressed the need for industrial health services, especially for adolescents.

These recommendations were made over sixty years ago and in England they met with a good deal of opposition from time to time, but most of them have gradually been put into action. The first advance was an Act for the prevention of cruelty to children and a general statute requiring school medical inspection in all public elementary schools—the first of the personal health services of a general character of this kind were not achieved without opposition; one example will suffice:

There was an appeal on behalf of a number of School Boards, recommending that meals should be provided for underfed children in school at the expense of the local taxes. The London newspaper, *The Times,* commented:

There is a section of the Board which aims at saddling upon the taxpayers all the responsibility for the feeding of the children sent to school without their proper meals, a policy which, we have contended from the first, will inevitably tempt a large class of parents to starve or half-starve their boys and girls in order to escape a burden to which they are legally subject and which they are very well able to bear.

Well, it was not true. Parents were not so cruel as *The Times* had suggested and, in fact, some years later when school meals were introduced, there was no trouble of this kind whatever.

REFERENCES

[1] HAMMOND, J. L. & BARBARA (1927): *The Village Labourer,* 4th ed., p. 308, London, Longmans.

[2] SMITH, SYDNEY (1804): *The Edinburgh Review,* May 4.

[3] SIMON, SIR JOHN, M.D. (1890): *English Sanitary Institutions,* p. 433, London, Cassell, 1890.

Chapter 2

HOSPITAL CARE

For in the circuit of the city . . . they have set four hospitals, so big, so wide, so ample, and so large, that they may seem four little towns, which were divised of that bigness partly to the intent the sick, be they never so many in number, should not lie too throng or strait, and therefore uneasily or incommodiously: and partly that they which were taken and holden with contagious diseases such as be wont by infection to creep from one to another, might be laid apart far from the company of the residue.

These hospitals be so well appointed, and with all things necessary to health so furnished, and moreover so diligent attendance through the continual presence of cunning physicians is given, that though no man be sent thither against his will, yet notwithstanding there is no sick person in all the city, that had not rather lie there than at home in his own house.*

In recent years, admittedly in the close confines of a city, it is necessary to construct many storeys, because of the high cost of land, but this should be looked on as an inevitable necessity rather than an ideal. Sir Thomas More speaks of the hospital as being in the circuit of the city, a little without the walls, and that is the ideal to be aimed at, even today, to avoid isolation of the patient, and even of the staff. Elaborate buildings of many storeys always carry the risk that the patient may be lost in a welter of machinery and elevators. He may be so far from the ground that he loses contact with it. In the bad old days of the English Poor Law, and indeed today in many countries, one of the prevailing criticisms against hospitals was that aged people were pushed up into a top storey, and never allowed out again because of the inconvenience of moving the bed. This is still a genuine risk even in the presence of elevators.

One of my most useful experiences in hospital administration was in Scotland, just before the onset of the second world war. We found that we were very short of beds for the accommoda-

* Sir Thomas More—Utopia.

tion of the astronomical number of casualties that had been estimated, and there was the additional difficulty that the great existing hospitals were all situated in vulnerable areas in the cities. We were therefore obliged to go outside the main centres of population, and to put up new hospitals in country sur-roundings. Naturally, we put up simple, one-storey buildings, and we laid stress on only two things: good heating and easy communication between one unit of the hospital and another. I think we failed in not providing sufficient centralised heating to make a thoroughly sound system, but at that time it was difficult to get elaborate engineering work done. We did, however, make the units sufficiently close to each other to provide for excellent communication by means of covered, enclosed roadways, which were also heated. At that time the pundits said: 'We suppose this hospital building is inevitable, but you realise you are putting up a lot of material which will be quite useless after the war, except perhaps as homes for mental defectives or store-houses for surplus war material'. Now as a matter of fact these simple units were a success from the start as acute general hospitals, and every bed provided at that time remained in occupation by the sick even in preference to the city hospitals. What were the reasons for success? It is not pos-sible to make a simple analysis. The first, oddly enough, is flexibility. The ward units were of standard size and were therefore easily interchangeable, and could be quickly adapted for any new purpose. I recollect, for example, a brain surgeon looking gloomily at one of these standard units and wondering how on earth he could treat patients effectively in such con-ditions. In a matter of a few weeks his unit was transformed in accordance with his own plans into a modern, fully air-condi-tioned brain surgery unit, with an operating room and all the diagnostic apparatus required by modern science. He was delighted. In the same way, a unit could be adapted quickly for one purpose and then changed for another, according to immediate needs; for example, a temporary outbreak of communicable disease, or an unexpected concentration of patients of a kind requiring highly specialised treatment.

We may describe a second reason for success in very simple terms as 'nearness to the ground'. It is strange how the great hospital which is built away up in the air tends to lose contact with the earth, and with the human beings who are going about their daily affairs. It becomes a kind of cloister—a reserved place where there is peace, without understanding. This is perfectly appropriate and proper for patients who are acutely ill or who require immediate surgery, but the ordinary patient who has a chronic disease, or who just suffers from the pangs associated with old age, is apt to feel lost away up there. This is equally true with convalescents. Down on the ground the patient knows how easy it is for visitors to come and go, without a sense of awe—a feeling that they have all been translated into some rarefied atmosphere. He knows that if the weather is warm and pleasant there is a real chance of getting out into the air and sun, and having a chat with friends under the trees. It is so easy to move a bed at ground level; pavilions, balconies and sun rooms are all very well, but they never give the same feeling of being in contact with the land.

The third point is simplicity. One cannot always assume that a new building of one storey will be cheaper to construct, because of the cost of land, although in the less developed areas this is undoubtedly so, but given sufficient land, one-storey buildings are easy to adapt, and it is always possible to add to them without great cost when some completely new provision is desired—as for the care of the mentally sick or the aged.

Mental patients particularly should receive their medical care close to the ground level, so that they have not the feeling of confinement which has been so common in the great mental hospitals of the past. The secret of success is imaginative transport arrangements, and simplicity, and compactness of construction.

In transport of supplies, the hospital of the future will show a great change. Since the distribution of supplies takes time, automation undoubtedly will play a larger part in simplifying supply items.

It is clear, however, that there are many hospitals today, especially in the developing countries, which go in for multi-storeyed buildings where there is no conceivable point for them. It has been suggested recently that there are five stages of patient care which together form a programme of continuing recovery.

1. An intensive care unit for the critically ill.
2. Intermediate care unit for patients whose condition has

become stabilised and no longer require active remedial care.

   3. A self-care unit of the hostel type for patients who are physically able to look after themselves, their only requirements being either restorative or diagnostic.

   4. A continuation care unit for long-term illness.

   5. An organised home care programme that is linked with hospital.

A great deal has been written recently in a number of countries about the system appropriately called Progressive Patient Care. As a result of this, the American Hospital Association invited a group of persons directly involved in this type of work to take part in a Symposium, which produced an excellent report on the subject in 1959.

As regards Mental Hospitals, the Minister of Health of that day, Mr. Powell, made this valid comment:—

> ... There comes a point where the very improvement of existing facilities militates powerfully against their supersession by something different and better. The resistance is not only physical. Hundreds of men and women, professional or voluntary, have given years, even lifetimes, to the service of a mental hospital or a group of mental hospitals.
>
> From such bodies it demands no mean moral effort to recognise that the institutions themselves are doomed. The transformation of the mental hospitals, continued the Minister, was not only a matter of buildings or the change of a physical pattern, it was also the transformation of a whole branch of the profession of medicine, of nursing, of hospital administration. Politics apart, everyone had a great deal of the conservative in his make-up, and found it easier to envisage things going on much as at present, than deliberately to choose and favour the unaccustomed and the drastic, and voluntarily to bring about a pattern of organisation in which new tasks would be performed in a new and wider setting.[1]

In England, the Mental Health Act of 1959 gave a clear direction to the change of attitude towards mental disorder, which has occurred not only in the health services but also in the general public. There has been a remarkable advance in their humanity and understanding since the middle of the century.

As early as 1935, the Board of Control was clearly aware of this change in attitude. Although they had not fully grasped at that time its effect on hospital construction, the Board took the point at any rate that institutional care is only a part of health service which includes all aspects of mental hygiene.

When a country is ripe for development, the first cry is usually for hospitals rather than for health services. A quarter of a century ago, when I was a member of the British Colonial Advisory Committee, we had occasion to ask a representative from Nigeria what he considered the first priority in their health service. 'A hospital', he replied, without a moment's hesitation. At that time I myself thought that this was the very negation of health, and I said so. But I have changed my mind as the years passed, without in the least degree losing my faith in the fundamental importance of a public health service in every area. Now I see more clearly that in a developing country you must begin with something that the people can see, some institution that performs 'miracles of healing', that supercedes the witch doctor. But that is not nearly all. You must begin with something that can be seen and visited—and understood—long before you attempt to send out feelers into the community. The building alone is not enough; it must contain people who are able and willing to teach, to help those who are in distress, and so to lead them eagerly towards health. They must first be convinced through sympathy and understanding what a *health* service means, and realise through practice the importance of prevention and of healthy living. The sore need of improved environment, with water supply and drainage, lurks in the background, while the presence of the sick is obvious. It is always the preventive attitude that has to be fostered by education. Eagerness for cure to the exclusion of prevention is natural in backward peoples. This early attitude is not so wrong as it sounds. A hungry generation seeks food before it is ready for instruction, and a sick people naturally clamours for the treatment of those who suffer, long before it is prepared to receive the doctrine of prevention. In one important respect they are quite right, because the best advertisement for health is the plain sight of someone being restored to health. As it happens, modern medicine armed with its syringe and its antibiotic wonders, is altering the whole picture. This is because it can demonstrate the effects of treatment without the old need for long hospital care, and often in the home itself, surrounded by sanitary conditions that would have shocked our ancestors. It is not going too far to say that in Russia today, many of the costly and long-established advances in environmental sanitation are being by-passed in the more urgent interests of immunisation and anti-biotic treatment. This attitude is equally true of many of the developing countries which have recently acquired their independence. One could easily be shown round a number of cities today that have gravely regressed in sanitation, but are retaining a substantial degree of health in a wilderness of neglected drains and watercourses. There are new towns where the discovery of some precious metal or other money-making find has brought about a great influx of work-hungry immigrants. They live in shacks and move around in a sea of ordure and empty food cans; but they live. And they have plenty of money by their standards.

Hospital services, especially through their out-patient departments, have ample opportunities for undertaking preventive measures. There is a close link, now widely recognised, between the prevention of sickness and the restoration to full health. In the modern hospital the patient is not merely a sick unit in bed; he is also a member of the community in which the hospital operates, and there is no true separation between the person at home, in work, or under medical care. The organisation of medical social work has brought this home to us.

The preventive services within the hospital may be briefly set out in the following groups:—

1. The laboratories. The recognised tests such as urine analysis, blood examination, and serological studies are among the oldest of preventive measures; but the work extends much further today, to include, for example, biopsy, blood culture, and prolonged functional studies under controlled conditions.

2. Radiological examinations now cover a wide range of preventive work, much of it applicable to the community at large. One may cite mass miniature photography, serial pictures, studies aimed at the prevention and early diagnosis of such conditions as tuberculosis and cancer, and also new investigations made necessary by the development of atomic energy, and a fresh assessment of the hazards of radiation.

3. Clinical examinations are becoming more and more preventive in character. Among the most important, from the

community point of view are nutritional studies, investigations of dietary disorders and deficiencies, and many tests of functional efficiency associated with modern medical and surgical treatment, and in the broader sense, with prevention.

4. Psychiatric investigations, as a means of prevention and early diagnosis, including the reaction of the patient to medical care. The building up of the patient's confidence is a matter of increasing importance, and in these times of stress the psychiatrist and his staff are often the most valuable links between hospital and home, between specialist and general practitioner.

5. Social work in the medical field brings out with growing intensity the fact that many patients have problems which grow in bulk under hospital conditions, partly because of the illness itself and partly because of the relative isolation of the patient from home surroundings. The mere fact that a person lies in bed in an institution—and this applies to maternity as well as sickness—often leads to brooding over difficulties that could easily be dispersed or overcome in ordinary circumstances. It is in these cases that the medical social worker can render incalculable service as an agent of prevention and the promotion of health.

6. Physiotherapy is often thought of as a means of restoring function to an injured limb or to a part of the body which has been damaged or immobilised by an illness. It may seem paradoxical to say so, but physiotherapy goes much farther than that—into the realm of psychotherapy. The injured limb is by no means the whole sickness. The physiotherapist is responsible, under medical supervision, for the maintenance of function and tone in the patient as a whole person. There are also enormous *psychological* benefits accruing to a sick, depressed patient from the physical care given in physical therapy. I often think that we do not appreciate this sufficiently, particularly with the long-term patient.

7. Hospital records are commonly regarded as matters of administrative convenience, but they render valuable aid in prevention. Properly handled, records are the basis for investigating groups of cases in both time and quantity in such a way that their study may well lead to the discovery of a new disease entity or a new method of treatment. Accurate records are instruments of modern hospital epidemiology; they are in-

valuable in the study of non-communicable diseases and for the scientific assessment of the relative value of different surgical procedures, or the follow-up on a long term basis of chronic illness with a view to adopting better methods of prevention and rehabilitation.

8. Research under hospital conditions is the essence of good medicine. Its range should cover all degrees from purely scientific research directed to the discovery of new knowledge to field studies in co-operation with general practitioners. In addition, one ought to bear in mind the value of social research in relation to the hospital services. Medicine today is a social as well as a physical science, and the way of progress is to link medicine with the disciplines of social science. The study of the patient against the background of home and family, work and play, interests and anxieties is of great assistance in discovering the factors which will help to relieve tension and promote the restoration of health.

9. In the field of pure administration there is abundant scope for research at the scientific level. The hospital services of today in all countries have to keep their house in order, and for this reason alone comparative studies are of great value. Administrators have to be constantly receptive of new methods of operation, other forms of financial and economic procedures, and other people's methods of financing hospital care.

10. So far I have been considering primarily the internal functions of the hospital service; but one of the most striking changes of the past few years has been the new attitude towards the external relations. In the modern hospital the work of the out-patient department has become the principal focus for all health activities.

Administration. In the health services of tomorrow there will be great scope for trained administrators, both medical and lay, and it is of the utmost importance that they learn to work together as a team. This has been foreseen in a number of countries and excellent courses of training in public administration and cognate subjects have already been established. Hitherto, the corresponding need for training medical men and women in administration has not been widely recognised, and doctors whose interests are mainly clinical have been slow to appreciate the value of administrative medicine or to realise that it is a proper and worthy career for medical practitioners whose talents lie in that direction. It is not surprising, therefore, that controversy has arisen from time to time over the respective spheres of medical and lay administration, largely because the scope of medical administration has not been defined with sufficient precision.

Medical administration extends into many fields, including institutions for the sick, the public health services, the industrial medical service, the growing social service, and the organisation of the medical profession itself. Some of these divisions obviously require special practical training and experience, which no purely academic course can provide. It follows that a large part of the training must be a practical 'apprenticeship'. Nevertheless, there are certain essential principles, and certain basic subjects of study which should be expounded by the academic teacher. These are common ground for postgraduate students in public health, industrial medicine, and general administration of institutions for the sick. They should be the foundations on which medical graduates can build their experience in any of the departments of administration. It would be unreasonable to expect a medical officer who is undergoing training to fit himself for medical practice to acquire, without special training and experience, the qualifications required of the administrator. This proposition will probably be generally accepted, but it would by no means justify a conclusion that medical administration should be handed over wholly to the layman. On the contrary, the right deduction to be drawn is that, as special training and practical experience are essential, they should therefore be provided forthwith in the form of a recognised study for medical men and women who wish to take up medical administration as a career. This applies particularly to those who are going abroad, and are taking part in the organisation of hospitals in the developing countries. The ordinary medical curriculum is the foundation upon which many careers are built. Practically all of these, such as surgery, gynecology, radiology, and public health require special training and practical experience before the graduate is qualified to follow his chosen path. Medical administration of tomorrow, whether in institution or in the field, stands in the same category.

Medical and lay administration ought not to be in conflict with each other; they are complementary, and both are necessary. The hospital, for example, is primarily an institution devoted to medical care, that is, the care of the sick, and its object is to restore them as far as possible to full health. The work of the medical administrator is to co-ordinate the services of a group of highly specialised medical scientists and other experts whose function coincides with the general aim of the institution. This demands an appreciation of the needs of such a service which can be best given by a man with basic medical training. Sometimes the idea has been fostered that the medical man is by that token an incompetent administrator, and even to propound the theory that medical training as such has an adverse effect on administrative ability. It is true that many general practitioners are individualists. There is no reason to suspect that this is a congenital defect, but it points clearly to the fact that training in administrative co-operation is essential. The hospital is, in addition, a business organisation. Its daily task in the community presents innumerable problems of business management, personnel and material, purchasing, finance and public relations. These problems offer abundant scope for the trained administrator. There is, for example, a constant need for internal control of the hospital's activities through an efficient accounting system, both costing and administrative records. Again, quite apart from the professional staff, every hospital of any size has a heavy load of domestic and technical staff, with all the organisation of a large hotel. Wage policies have to be decided; food has to be cooked and served to the satisfaction of residents and guests, many of the latter being involuntarily more difficult about their diet than the average hotel guest; and finally, non-professional 'bedroom-service' has to be given to an extent far greater than in most hotels. It is a fantastic anomaly that food service as opposed to supervision of diet should be carried out by trained nurses. It is equally wrong that catering, purchasing, accountancy, and non-professional management should be undertaken by a medical man. On the other hand, medical care in its broadest sense—the health of the hospital and its inmates—is clearly a medical function and should not be delegated either to the layman or the casual physician. The need here is for team-work and such subjects as medical and nursing equipment and services, the organisation of professional staff, and the various departments in which they work, require a team consisting at least of medical and lay administration and the principal nurse to serve its primary function of making the sick whole, and of bringing comfort to those who are anxious and distressed, whether they be patients or their relatives.

Dr. Bradley[2] made an excellent summary of the situation:—

> The hospital can be viewed as a living organism whose chief anatomical components or parts are living beings, some working, some learning, some residing, some receiving treatment, all in a group environment and under one roof. The hospital has many characteristics of a living person. We can properly call it a biosocial organism.

ENEMIES OF THE PATIENT

Quite recently I was in a hospital where administrative efficiency had run mad. The patient was described officially as 'a unit of sickness'. Even in more humane hospitals, however, it is not a good thing to be a patient, unless one is ill. I once knew a man who was convalescent and he was able to move around fairly well in a large, crowded ward. I understand that he was mistaken for a ward attendant for several months! The story is also told of a young surgical intern who was believed to be a patient because of his diffidence in the wards. It is easy to tell when a patient is ill: he is either silent or he bleats like a little ewe lamb. When he becomes difficult and cantankerous, he is convalescent.

The patient in bed has enemies lurking amongst his many real friends in hospital. The first and greatest of these is:

NOISE. He must be able to open and close his ears at will. In consideration of the noise going on by day and by night in many hospitals he will be tempted to keep them permanently closed. The main elements of this more or less constant hubbub are:—

Lifts. These are called 'elevators' in America. They are so designed as to create the greatest possible noise over the largest possible area. Their gates clang, with a jangle of discord; the machinery, although housed far away in the basement, uses the shaft to trumpet its mechanical faults at all times, and finally the lift is placed as close as possible to the patient area.

Movable furniture. This consists of quite a number of things on squeaky wheels used to carry food or medical equipment and dressings or even (in the more primitive hospitals) a pestilent substance called coal. There are many ways of making a noise with these trolleys. Perhaps the most effective and loudest is to bang them against doorposts and beds. Another successful method is to place cups, saucers, etc. on them in such a way that they rattle violently with every movement. Bed screens on wheels can be designed to give excruciating agony to sensitive patients. Even curtains on rails can be so maintained as to give constant irritation when they are moved on their runners.

Other human beings in the hospital. Some of the noises cannot be altogether avoided: there are, for example, patients who are noisy by nature or illness: and there are those dear souls who carry on a conversation about their children or grandchildren across the ward. Unnecessary noise created by the staff is sometimes a just cause for complaint. Laughter and cheerfulness on part of nurses and attendants are great assets, but their ministrations can be overdone in the late evening; and then there is the house surgeon who arrives on the ward at 2 a.m. after having had a pleasant evening at the local pub.

Noises outside. In a newspaper I came across this letter from the Administrator and Secretary of one of the largest teaching hospitals in London. It is interesting and significant:

HOSPITAL NOISE

You carried two letters last week from patients complaining of the noise made by cars and motorcycles starting up in the streets round this hospital. My Board of Governors are greatly concerned about this nuisance as they are well aware that this goes on until the small hours of the morning. Everyone realises that this must be particularly trying for patients, but unfortunately the authorities who are responsible for controlling our parking places are not influenced by these considerations.

About two years ago the police sited public parking places alongside the hospital and, in reply to our protest, informed us that it would practically take an Act of Parliament to have these parking places moved a short distance away from the hospital.

Our problem would be greatly eased if a short section of the road at the back of the hospital could be turned into a private roadway and thereby closed at night. This is being considered at present by the local authority.

T. F. W. Mackeown,
Administrator and Secretary,
University College Hospital,
St. Pancras.

Evening Standard, 12.1.53.

EXCESSIVE LIGHT

He must be able to dim or black-out his eyes at will. There is nothing more trying for a patient who is sick in bed than a bright light full in his eyes. This may come from a window by day or a ceiling light by night. There is in England a historical reason for our failure to appreciate the importance of design in lighting. Years ago hospitals were stuffy, dangerous and full of smells. The sanitarians of the late nineteenth century were naturally anxious about light and ventilation and in hospital design they went to the extreme worship of cubic space. They provided enormous windows, ceilings of incredible height, and bright, draughty wards. These one can see today in almost any large general hospital. The ceilings are so high in fact that some of the four-bed rooms would be considerably more commodious if they were laid on their side. These sick rooms may be agreeable to visitors and even nurses and they lend a certain dignity to the view; but they are very annoying to patients, especially the unfortunate people who are fixed in frames or other apparatus. In most of our new or redesigned hospitals the beds are placed side-ways to the windows and that is all to the good because it gives much more freedom to the patient and helps him to get away from the light, but how are we to improve the innumerable older hospitals where these changes are hardly possible? Outside blinds and shutters may give some relief but they tend to cover too great a window area. We often provide movable screens for patients out of doors and the principle of the adjustable shade which could be moved by the patient himself would be of value indoors also, especially when the bright light is shining on the bed.

Another method is to grow eyebrows sufficiently large, dark and bushy to act as eyeshades. This saves the hospital the trouble and expense of doing anything about it.

LACK OF PRIVACY

This enemy appears in several forms, some material and others like malignant ghosts. When a patient lies in an open ward, especially if this has more than four beds, he must, if he is at all sensitive, feel the need at some time of the day to be by himself. A large room means that everything has to be shared by everybody, that every action may be seen by prying eyes. Movable screens, although useful for toilet and dressing purposes, do not meet the patient's real need for a little privacy. Probably the best method is to have curtains with fixed rails above each bed so that the patient can himself draw the curtains, partly or wholly, if only to screen himself from neighbouring occupants. This is little protection against noise but it at least cuts off excessive light and the irritating feeling of constant movement.

Another enemy is that abominable anachronism known as the bed-pan. We are learning at last in many hospitals, in the interest of safety, quiet and efficiency, to provide special rooms for dressings and other personal attentions to patients. We have yet to learn in most hospitals that special rooms provided with toilet and lavatory basin are essential for the comfort for all but a few patients. There are, of course, emergencies and exceptional cases which have to be met but in the overwhelming majority, patients are far less exhausted and far more comfortable when they can be taken to an appropriately designed lavatory for washing and toilet.

In a very real sense this is an engineering problem rather than a medical or architectural one and it is high time we invited the engineer to advise us. I have never been able to understand why in hospital design and management we are so reluctant to put the fundamental problems of *lifting* and *moving* to the engineer and bring him into our counsels. We are in the absurd position that in industry we can easily, almost without effort, lift one or a dozen wooden cases weighing 300 pounds apiece; but we still lack a design for lifting and moving a patient weighing perhaps 150 pounds or less. Modern methods of simple weight-raising apparatus should be studied and applied to the patient in bed. When that has been done the special room will replace the bed-pan for the vast majority of patients and for mechanical lifting of a sick person a much more efficient apparatus, anatomically and physiologically, will meet the patient's needs at the bedside.

LONELINESS

So far I have been quoting a few illustrations dealing only with the physical side of a patient's needs but, of course, that is not nearly enough; there are many enemies with much greater subtlety in the psychological field. I think we should speak first perhaps about loneliness. Most people who are no longer acutely ill feel that time goes rather slowly. On the other hand they are often quickly fatigued by conversation and also by frequent interference for one service and another. Even where visitors are most welcome, patients in hospital are easily tired by the effort of talking and of concentrating their minds on matters outside the hospital routine. Half an hour should be the maximum for a visitor. On the other hand, it is notorious that many patients, adults as well as children, in single rooms are apt to become desperately lonely and miserable. Loneliness is an enemy, but excessive attention, fussiness and interference are almost as vicious. The ideal is to strike a balance between the two according to the patient's needs and wishes. It is sometimes not realised that a patient can be as lonely in a crowded ward as in a separate room.

In many cases patients are worried by lack of a reasonably continuous period for sleep. It has been said bitterly that a patient's working hours in hospital are from 4 a.m. to 10 p.m. and this indictment is true enough where there are innumerable petty services, examinations and consultations to prevent the patient having continuity of rest. This problem deserves close study at regular intervals in every nursing unit. Another serious enemy to the patient's wellbeing in hospital is a sense of insecurity: this is partly due to doubt about the course of the illness but even more often to the lack of somebody to sit down and answer simple questions from time to time. In one of our leading newspapers not very long ago there was a good deal of correspondence about the anxiety that patients feel before an operation or a confinement and a number of patients complained that if only some kindly person had told them what to expect, it would have made all the difference to their comfort and relieved any apprehension. This is by no means always the fault of the administrative services in the hospital. There is in England, at any rate, a long tradition of silence amounting to secrecy about medical matters. We should give more study to the question of what a patient should be told. The facile attempts to allay fears by telling nothing in soothing words is a greater irritation to most patients than mere silence. Patients do not like to be treated like small children; and incidentally even small children need some words of explanation before anything happens to them in hospital.

In all my enquiries about patient amenities I have been struck again and again by complaints about the conduct of confinements in hospital. One young mother after another has told me plaintively that she was left alone and in fear about the time of the delivery of the child. I am satisfied on enquiry that the overwhelming majority of these complaints are due to a misunderstanding which could easily be cleared up when the mother has recovered from the immediate effects of labour. If I am right what seems to happen is this: that towards the end of the second stage the patient, who is in any case in pain and discomfort, is given an anaesthetic of one kind or another. Even the mildest anaesthesia is sufficient for considerable disorientation; the patient no longer sees clearly the people who are around her and she imagines that she is entirely alone. Very often some kind of explanation is given before the baby is born and the surgeon or nurse says comfortingly 'I will be with you at the time'. In spite of this, apprehension quickly turns to resentment when she goes over her experiences after the baby is born. Now if someone were to sit beside her for a few minutes and explain in clear enough language what happened and say 'I was there' then her apprehension and resentment would be quickly dissolved and so we should be relieved of many uncessary complaints.

Many volumes on the qualities of a good administrator have been issued, and it might be valuable to study the qualities of a good patient for a change.

1 A patient's education should conform to the standards established by the American College. He should be conversant with the current trends of medical treatment and thoroughly posted on everything pertaining to the sickroom.

2. He should have a pleasant personality and so inspire confidence in his medical and nursing attendants.

3. Sense of importance. He must be mindful of the fact that he is the person about whom the entire institution revolves and that his own comfort comes first.

4. Tact and diplomacy. Probably no vocation, other than being a patient requires more tact and discretion in handling people. There are nurses to be considered and attendants who bring tepid meals, often poorly served; there is the need for affability during the farce of the consultant's weekly round at the head of a column of lesser personages. A colleague of mine, himself recently in hospital, said, 'The patient is so over-awed that he asks none of the questions he would like to, and even if he did it is doubtful if he would get a reasonable answer'. The cultivated air of detachment is not reassuring to the patient who has after all some interest in his illness and deserves a little recognition in any discussion round the bedside.

5. Patience. This is obviously the basic need of the patient. There is little to be gained, and much to be lost, by throwing the bed-pan out of the window.

6. A controlled sense of humour. The patient may find considerable scope for entertainment but when the matron, or principal nurse, slips on a discarded banana skin his laughter should not be too obvious.

7. A sense of fairness. You cannot be a good patient unless you can see your position in relation to the staff and the other patients.

These are merely light illustrations but you will appreciate that they conceal a good deal of serious thought beneath. The administrator's main duty to patients, I feel, is to make sure that they have a sense of confidence in the hospital and all of its staff. This can be done by careful education and explanation before unusual or frightening events occur and when a sick person has to undergo an operation it is of vital importance to tell him about it and to say in Browning's words:

You will wake, and remember, and understand.

REFERENCES

[1]POWELL, E. (1961): National Association for Mental Health, *Brit. med. J.*, 18th Mar., p. 820.
[2]BRADLEY, F. R. (1959): Trends in hospital administration, *Hospital (N.Y.)*, August.

Chapter 3

THE STATE AND THE CHILD

BOSWELL: 'If, Sir, you were shut up in a castle, and a new-born child with you, what would you do?'

JOHNSON: 'Why, Sir, I should not much like my company.'

BOSWELL: 'But would you take the trouble of rearing it?'

JOHNSON: 'Why yes, Sir, I would; but I must have all conveniences. If I had no garden, I would make a shed on the roof, and take it there for fresh air. I should feed it, and wash it much, and with warm water to please it, not with cold water to give it pain.'

BOSWELL: 'But, Sir, does not heat relax?'

JOHNSON: 'Sir, you are not to imagine the water is to be very hot. I would not *coddle* the child.'

This subject is of special importance on account of its early and continuing international significance. It would be idle to attempt to assess exact priorities for the care of mother and child, but it is evident that this was from the beginning of the missionary movement one of the first and foremost medical tasks. Wherever the gospel was preached among the poorer or more primitive races, there the protection of mother and child became a primary concern. This is not surprising, because the appeal is great on both sides, and child care has the highest authority in the gospel story. Even today, if one were to ask a public health nurse what she regarded as her 'key to the home' she would be likely to answer 'The presence of a young child'. A more rigid attitude might have shadowed the missionary spirit before the scientific age; one sometimes feels that the injection of dogma may have preceded the attention to bodily needs. This is by no means fanciful, even in my lifetime. Many years ago I was medical officer to a number of infant welfare centres in a rural area. They were always run by voluntary organisations and as a rule the actual meetings were held in a church hall. I remember being asked on one occasion to give an address on infant care at a mothers' meeting. Half mischievously I enquired whether it mattered if I was a member of that particular faith, and I was surprised to be told that it made all the difference.

Half a century ago there were quite a number of voluntary societies directing their efforts specially to the care of the mother and child. Many of these were known as 'home missions' and I gather that the name was taken in contrast to the 'foreign missions' which were earlier in time. The main purpose of these missions was to bring religious belief to backward people, whether at home or abroad; but it was not long before the enlightened missionaries found that they could not teach religion effectively unless they did something to relieve the gross poverty, superstition and ignorant neglect from which families suffered, both at home and abroad, in the nineteenth century. This is not a very old story, in rural England at any rate. When just after the end of the first world war I took up a post as an assistant health officer, I found to my surprise that my chief opponent was the local witch, to whom hundreds of people flocked at the week-ends—for her cottage was not very accessible, and the mothers had often to take long walks with their children to reach this fount of knowledge. The local medical practitioners, on the other hand, were almost invariably kindly, if a trifle contemptuous of the school medical service, and in many cases this gentle contempt was justified by their wisdom and seniority, and the fact that they, and they alone, were giving continuity of medical care. As time went on their friendliness increased and we often found occasion for consultation, in which I learned a great deal about the clinical aspects, but was able to tell them about the social aspects—for example, the social care of a child suffering from long-term illness or a condition requiring prolonged orthopaedic treatment. (Half a generation later, as a more senior health officer, I was frequently consulted on the diagnosis and disposal of patients suspected of a notifiable infectious disease. In return for this, the school medical officer received steadily increasing help from the local practitioners in supporting advice given at the clinics to the mothers.)

Before the end of the nineteenth century, as we have seen, the cause of environmental sanitation in Europe, and especially in Germany and the Scandinavian countries, had won a resounding victory with the introduction of effective sanitary legislation. Some time before the close of the century a broad advance had been made towards the conception of *personal* health, or at least towards removing some of the worst obstructions that lay in its path. The value of the individual and his family, and the importance of the child in the community, was being impressed on the state in various ways, mainly through the rise of clinics for infant feeding, as in France. The most prominent of these movements deserves the title of a 'social revolution'. Progress was all the more steady because it was both scientific and practical, in the sense that it won the support of many types of opinion and belief. At this time many social organisations turned up material for reform by legislation, and it is not surprising that the most prominent of these were linked with the work of women who were beginning to find their independence and value in the world of social advance.

One of the earliest schemes for improving the health of children was the system which originated in Switzerland of organising holiday colonies. This idea spread rapidly over Europe and reached Russia by the end of the nineteenth century. The funds for plans of this kind were collected by a local voluntary committee during the winter months. The head teacher sent in the names of the most deserving children—the poor and weakly, but not actually sick. The children were usually sorted into groups of ten to fifteen under a single teacher and were sent into the country for a month or so during the school holidays.

In England, the official effort to promote the health of mothers and children begins appropriately with the first Midwives Act in the year 1902. In general, voluntary efforts had different origins and many of them arose independently in various parts of the country and for a long time proceeded along their own lines. Often a special movement sprang up to deal with one objective, such as midwives, or the provision of care for the new-born. As time went on these movements began to get together. They had been travelling towards the same destination but along different paths, and the time came when the agencies that had worked in isolation began to co-ordinate. The maternity and child welfare movement is the result of many voluntary efforts along these lines. In one way it

is peculiar, because owing to missionary leadership its international phase in undeveloped countries in some respects
preceded the national movements among the more advanced
countries.

It is always difficult to assign a definite beginning to any
social movement. Each has its forerunners in isolated local
attempts to remove obvious evils. A local society is often founded by one person or a little group. As it becomes more widely
known it stimulates efforts in other localities. The movement
for the protection of mothers and their infants had its local
forerunners in the eighteenth century in the provision of
maternity hospitals. It was about that time that the Foundling
Hospital stimulated interest in the neglected child. In the
nineteenth century child care gradually developed in relation
to the restriction of child labour in factories and workshops, but
very little was done for the broader maternity and child welfare
movement. This was a social force that ultimately drew public
attention to the evils that faced child life and development,
and showed that carefully administered Acts of Parliament
could do much to protect the more helpless members of society.
Broadly speaking, the maternity and child welfare movement
was the result of agitation to protect the foster child, which
began in the second half of the nineteenth century. The Infant
Life Protection Society was founded in 1870 and achieved
success by the passing of an Act in 1872 which was the first of a
long series. Next came the movement for the recognition of
midwives, which began with the investigation of child mortality
undertaken in 1867 by the Obstetrical Society of London on the
initiative of William Farr.

The infant welfare movement as such is really a product of the
twentieth century. At that time the continuance of a high rate
of infant mortality was becoming a matter of serious public
concern. It seemed a curious setback to the movements for
sanitary reform which had achieved success in other respects
during the preceding fifty years. During this period infant
mortality showed no decline, and indeed seemed to be rising
at the end of the century. At this time England was by no
means the only country contemplating with some anxiety a
high mortality rate in infants combined with a falling birth
rate. This was of special concern in France, and it was there

that an Infant Consultation and Milk Depot was first established. Almost at the same time a school for mothers was set up in Belgium, and here we see the essential feature of child welfare work—that in order to help the child we must teach mothercraft. This is the germ of all fully developed maternal and child health centres.

The next movement was obvious enough to those who were becoming interested in this work. It was necessary to keep in touch with the children who had been brought to the infant welfare centres and to find out what was happening in those homes from which the children were *not* brought to the centres. At first, this visiting was done by voluntary workers, mostly untrained middle-class women who were interested in children and anxious to help—but it was soon found that more skilled and more regular supervision was necessary. In this way the public health nurse came into being in many districts. In some cases home visiting came before the establishment of infant welfare centres, and indeed stimulated that development. The earlier workers had the drawback of not knowing where the babies were, but this was gradually removed by the compulsory notification of births, which in England took place in 1915. In 1918 the first general Maternity and Child Welfare Act laid down the broad outline upon which all child welfare work in the United Kingdom is now based.

Our increasing knowledge of normal child development has enabled abnormalities to be detected at an earlier stage. Special toddlers' sessions have much improved our experience of the needs of handicapped children and have generally afforded an opportunity for earlier preventive treatment.

The falling death rate among new-born infants has been to some extent paralleled by an increased survival rate among handicapped children. In general, if these children are to make the best of their potentialities they should be reared in their own homes. This raises a number of family problems involving the parents, the child himself, and his brothers and sisters. Many of these problems are practical and others have their roots in difficult personal relationships, and it often takes a long time for doctors and case workers to assist the families to get them straightened out. It is of primary importance that a child's deviation from normal, either mentally or physically,

C

should be recognised as early as possible, and the nature of his handicap fully assessed. Where this is done at a clinic or hospital the medical officer of health is responsible for ensuring that treatment and training are arranged, and that the appropriate home visiting is regularly carried out. In many areas a special register of handicapped children is now kept, and the responsibility for a regular review of the cases devolves upon the senior medical officer. This important duty cannot be delegated to non-medical staff, even if the child is receiving treatment in hospital.

In the beginning it is often found that the parents need a simple explanation of the cause of the handicap, so that they will not suffer anxiety that they themselves are in some way to blame, or that the child is a victim of professional neglect. When they have recovered from the first shock they become ready to plan and to think in terms of the child's assets rather than his disabilities. The experience of most workers in this field is that unless the parents are skilfully guided to realise that the handicapped child will show all the instincts, drives and rebellions of the normal child, as well as the frustrations of his particular condition, they will fail to understand his often difficult and contradictory behaviour.

A few parents will accept their handicapped child with a matter of fact affection from the beginning. The majority tend to treat the child with over-protection or over-stimulation, and even in some cases with rejection. The tendency to over-protect is the commonest, and is a severe disadvantage in later life, because the child has never been taught to accept the inevitable frustrations of daily living. Over-pressure is less common, but is especially dangerous because it means very often that the parents are unwilling to accept the truth and are determined to prove that their child has the capacity to succeed as well as any normal child. The result of course is excessive nervousness and a tendency to withdraw in order to seek refuge. Regular home visiting and advice can do much to help. Total rejection is rare, but where the disabilities are such as those caused by the recent notorious cases of thalidomide poisoning, it is likely to become more common.

The Changing Need in Maternal and Child Health Centres

Since 1952 there has been a trend towards changing the routine of ante-natal and child welfare centres. From that date the ante-natal care of domiciliary cases showed that an increasing number of general practitioners were providing this care for their own booked cases. More general practitioners are now undertaking these responsibilities and to an increasing extent see their own patients, either at the surgery, often with the help of a midwife, or at the local maternal and child welfare centre; or they may themselves act as medical officers at the centre on a sessional basis. Interim care is given at a growing number of midwife sessions in the clinics, and more and more expectant mothers attend mothercraft and relaxation classes. In addition, an increasing number of local health authorities have appointed obstetricians to take care of consultant work, so that in some clinics there is now a team which may consist of general practitioner, midwife, health visitor and social worker or other member of the local authority staff, as required. This type of medical supervision has gradually increased, but it is still at a kind of experimental stage. The whole time assistant medical officer may be replaced by a general practitioner obstetrician in time, but in the meantime she continues in many areas to give full antenatal care, or she may provide supervision as an interim arrangement.

Ante-natal clinics still distribute welfare foods and maternity packs. Vaccination against poliomyelitis is now offered to expectant mothers, but the acceptance rate is only twenty per cent. The majority of those attending these clinics expect to be confined at home, but hospital-booked cases may attend for interim care. Applications for admission to hospital for social need is frequently made through the clinic.

Child Welfare Clinics

Changes have been varied—some clinical and some administrative. Clinics for healthy infants continue to function, and a high proportion of mothers bring their infants regularly to them during the first year. Recently there has been an increase in children between one and two years, but relatively few of that age attend with any regularity. Medical advice in the child welfare clinics is given mainly by full time medical officers, a growing number of whom hold joint appointments for maternal and child health and school health. General practitioners, however, are now taking an increasing number of sessions. This has the advantage that many full-time assistant medical officers are becoming more aware of the importance of keeping in touch with the family doctor and referring cases to him for appropriate action. Health visitors continue to be the mainstay of the clinic staff. Their association with general practitioners is improving and they are beginning to form a more important link between the clinic and the home, the family doctor, and sometimes the hospital.

Additional special sessions have been established, especially in connection with mental health. Some attention is being paid to backward babies and to spastics, and general guidance is given to parents on psychiatric grounds. At some of the special sessions the clinic's medical and nursing staff are brought into contact with specialists. This is especially important in audiology and in orthopaedics. Paediatric consultant sessions of a more general kind are held in a few areas, and in some cases the paediatrician also takes child welfare sessions.

Preventive Care

Viewed as a whole, there has been better appreciation in recent years of mental health and emotional factors, and the inter-relation between these and physical health. Some local authorities have in fact appointed a child psychiatrist, and in a few areas he also advises the mother directly; but the general pattern is for him to hold case conferences at which the medical and health visitor staff discuss their cases and seek guidance from the psychiatrist on how to deal with them.

The Ill Child in Hospital

A Committee in England published in 1959 a report on the welfare of the ill child in hospital. While it is difficult to summarise a report of this kind, there are certain recommendations which have a wide significance in relation to international health. In general, they felt that greater attention has to be paid to the emotional and mental needs of the child in hospital. The authority and responsibility of parents, the individuality of the child and the means of mitigating the effects of the break with home should all be more fully recognised. The Committee laid great stress on the measures required to reduce to a minimum the effect of removing a child from his parents and from the family background. This meant consideration of the child's emotional needs while in hospital, especially when he encounters conditions similar to those of the deprived child, with the added possibility of painful and frightening experiences. For this reason the Committee emphasised the value of admitting the mother with the young child under five wherever possible, and recommended that unrestricted visiting should be adopted by all hospitals. In this way the continuity of the child's way of life would be preserved. In general, children should not be admitted to hospital if this can be avoided, or only when the medical treatment they require cannot be given in other ways. When the nature of the illness and the home conditions permit, the mother should be encouraged to nurse her sick child at home under the care of the family doctor, preferably with the assistance of the district nurse.

The report of this Committee has not gone unchallenged. For example, a paediatrician writing in *The Guardian* on 21 November 1962, says:

> Why has there arisen, recently, this urge on the part of mothers to visit their children at all times? And why particularly by *literate* mothers? Because literate women read, and are influenced by what they read. There has recently been a spate of articles dealing with the dark dangers lurking about a child who has been admitted to hospital. Most such women now feel a deep sense of guilt when they allow—even for the most compelling reasons—their child to leave them. The mothers have been thoroughly frightened by an inflated bogy-man; from my own experience I am sure the picture has been exaggerated. Most paediatricians are well aware of children's emotional problems and cater for them.

In writing this he rather feels that the mainspring behind the mother's desire to be with the child in hospital is *her own need* to see the child, to reassure herself that all is well in that 'dreadful' place; and the greater the sacrifice in order to do this, the more is her conscience assuaged.

Finally, the paediatrician pleads for a sense of proportion. A few years ago, the visiting of the sick child was confined to a grudging afternoon a week. Many medical and nursing staff were not satisfied with that, and worked for more visiting; three or four times a week, and now daily. That, he feels, is appropriate and beneficial, but the pendulum continues to swing: **not** only every day, but *all* day, and all night too. In essence it is proposed that parents should camp in the hospital.

There is another comment from a mother whose child, a boy of 22 months, was admitted to hospital for a major operation. She arrived at the hospital with her child, determined to stay as long as he needed her. At this particular hospital every mother was given ample opportunity to settle her child into the ward, and no suggestion was ever made that they should leave. Feeding, washing, undressing—all were left to the mother if she wanted to do them. Then the hospital staff arranged for a bed for the mother, and she found herself one of a little group. For the first two days she was on the ward at 6.30 a.m. to see her child and spend all day with him, except for going out for her own meals. The last visit of the day was made at about 10 p.m., when she had a word with the night nurse. The boy was sound asleep, and had been so for hours. In fact, he settled in wonderfully, and loved the company of the other children. However, the testing time was yet to come. On the day of the operation the mother asked if she could be with William until he was 'asleep', and be there when he came back from the operating theatre. This is not advised, the Sister said, but if you want to be there, by all means. And stay there she did. The mother comments further: 'William was sound asleep before being lifted on to the trolley—he did not even stir. Where was the point in going any farther with him? So I went and had some coffee instead and was back on the ward when he returned from the theatre. It was at this point that I had to revise all my former opinions of whether Mum should be there or not.'

The mother here explains that before marriage she was a nurse, and that she is the wife now of a country doctor. She is used to ill people, hospitals, blood transfusions, and she believed herself to be an unemotional person. She was therefore totally unprepared for her reaction. She felt the most primitive maternal instinct welling up in her, and she wanted to snatch up the little body there on the trolley—blood bottles, tubes and all— and rush off with it. She felt that she was going to cry, and in fact she had to take herself off to a quiet place to take hold of

herself. Eventually, on returning to the ward, she found a peace-
fully sleeping child. He did wake up once or twice but made no
sign of noticing her or anyone else. For 24 hours or more he just
slept with an occasional few minutes awake for a wash or a
nappy change. 'In fact', comments the mother 'I should have
taken the Sister's advice and stayed away. Think of the upset
to all the children if I had been even a little more emotional
than I am or even less used to the sometimes alarming contrap-
tions that patients have attached to them after an operation.'
This letter concludes with the summing up:

> On reflection I think that daily visiting is essential—certainly
> for the under fives. And most hospitals will agree with this if the
> mother can conduct herself calmly all the time. Sleeping by the
> bedside is unnecessary both for the mother and the child. But
> by far the best guide is the ward sister. The one we had was a
> shrewd and experienced woman. She cannot afford to become
> sentimental or emotionally involved in all the pathetic little
> creatures who come under her care. Take a cue from her and make
> the whole 'ordeal' a matter-of-fact everyday business. Then your
> child will come through it feeling that is just what it has been.

PLAY SPACE FOR YOUNG CHILDREN

In the home of today it is of more than passing interest to
note that the provision of a play space has become a recognised
feature of child care, even from early infancy. The play pen is
an institution. It has come into being partly in response to the
growing difficulty of obtaining constant adult supervision of
babies, but mainly because it has been found in practice such a
valuable means of preventing a baby from doing itself harm.
The hazards of the home have increased in modern times with
the use of electricity and gas for a multitude of household
purposes, some of which are not free from risk. Quite apart
from this, there are more positive reasons for the popularity of
the play pen; it offers the child a little world of its own, and its
wooden walls are a source of constant interest. It is essential,
however, that the play-pen should be associated with pleasure
rather than hunger and misery.

When the child begins to move about on his feet, the pen is
no longer a barrier but a toy to be pushed around the room,
and it may reach dangerous corners. Be that as it may, the
child who has reached his feet needs more opportunities for

exploration. Activity and curiosity are now his main characteristics, and the harassed mother must give him ample scope for
their exercise. There is no escape. The mother and the family
have to conduct each child through the well-known 'No, no'
period up to the end of the second year at least.

One of the most important developments in our knowledge of
children during the past generation is, as Bowlby pointed out
'the steady growth of evidence that the quality of parental care
which a child receives in his earliest years is of vital importance
for his future mental health'. It is widely agreed that the critical
period for parental care to be effective is under three years.
During this period of a child's life the finest playground is the
garden at home, and in this respect the new estates of small
houses have much to offer. In some cases unfortunately the
garden attached to the home, when well cared for, becomes a
showplace rather than a play space, and there is not enough
freedom for the small child. The family garden may carry too
many restrictions and too few opportunities. In other cases,
especially when the families are housed in apartments, there
may be no defined garden space, thus allowing toddlers to roam
at will and get into mischief and even danger. One of the
remedies for this is to set up specially designed play spaces for
young children near their home. These spaces should provide a
hard surface on which small children can play with their toys
or run scooters and baby cars. Simplicity is the keynote. There
is no need for equipment in the form of swings and roundabouts,
or even sandpits. A plain shelter with a concrete roof on one
side of the space, with a bench of the same material inside, would
give the children protection against showers and cold winds,
and at the same time allow the mothers to rest awhile on their
way home from shopping while the younger children paddle
around with their mobile toys. This does not imply that the
toddler would always be under the mother's eye, but nearness
to home and safety from road traffic are part of a good playground scheme. It is a good plan to divide the play area irregu-
larly by constructing low walls of brick or concrete, as young
children greatly enjoy piloting their way along such walls. The
advantages of breaking up the space in this way are that it adds
interest for the toddlers themselves, and at the same time prevents older children from using the area for rough ball games

cycling or roller skating. In small play spaces of this kind there is no point in providing grass, shrubs and flowers. Grass is quickly turned to mud and thrown about, and shrubs and flowers do not survive unless they are planted in large clumps or otherwise protected.

In the development of shopping centres and supermarkets the provision of play spaces of this kind solves many problems for the hard pressed mother on her errands. These hard-surfaced play areas help to keep little children off streets and roadways which are traffic laden and dangerous. Although for the time being traffic in the newly-built estates is not of the city type, it is becoming increasingly fast and heavy. The number of automobiles per household is rising each year, as is shown by the fact that the present target for garage accommodation even in England is already one for every three houses, and this is now being regarded as a minimum. The chief objection of householders to these play-spaces is noise, and many tenants would rather have a garage. Both play spaces and garages are required, and this is a false alternative. Many planners suggest that there should be a space for play within a quarter of a mile of every dwelling in a built up area. The right size must be subject to experiment, but a quarter of an acre has been suggested as a minimum. There should be no elaborate fencing of the play space, but safety measures are necessary to prevent children from careering on to a thoroughfare.

THE PRE-SCHOOL CHILD

This period of childhood, which lies between the second and the fifth year, tends to be overlooked in many countries, even in those which are well advanced in infant care. The reasons are complex, but one thing that is certain is that the mother would welcome more help and advice. Her difficulty often is that if she has a younger child than the toddler she is unable to attend the infant welfare centre, and so she loses the double benefit. Maternal and child welfare clinics too find difficulty in getting competent help for looking after toddlers while the mother is engrossed with the new baby, and so the pre-school child gets the worst of both worlds. Unfortunately the young child has to face psychological difficulties of his own at the same time, on account of jealousy of the interposing baby, and often shows his feelings by conduct that only accentuates the hardship on the mother—by refusing food, whining, and general unwillingness to leave his mother's skirts. This, of course, is common knowledge, and many other psychological phenomena are described to account for the 'difficult age'. The net result, however, is that this age group tends to be nobody's business, and we are in the presence, in many cases, of what could be described as the dark age of childhood, just at the very time when bad habits are most likely to be formed, and when the common infections are apt to cause serious trouble to health and even life.

One of the obvious results of this is that the mother's attendance at the infant welfare centre is likely to drop off at this most important stage. A useful remedy is for the public health nurse to increase the number of her home visits when there is a toddler in the house, especially if another child has been born in the interval. It is important also that there should be a good hospital service for this age group, with little waiting time for attention and prompt arrangements for transportation. One of the well known hazards of this age group is that the children are apt to go down rapidly unless they receive prompt, skilled attention. They also respond badly and quickly to nutritional faults and are highly susceptible to gastro-intestinal infections. There is every reason to believe that one of the greatest single advances in medical services for children in the advancing countries is the appointment of nursing staff with a sound knowledge of nutrition and a capacity for dealing promptly with the common disorders of the pre-school age.

Quantity versus Quality

There are certain real difficulties in creating and maintaining services for children in the developing countries, although most of these can be sorted out in time. The first trouble is to arrange priorities when finances are limited, perhaps to a grant from a voluntary body. Should one go all out for quality, hoping for the best as time goes on through increasing contributions? If this is the policy it may be argued that one small section of the population is being given a benefit that should have been more fairly distributed. On the other hand, if quantity is preferred on the ground of fairness to all, then the sacrifice may be too great

—that is, an inferior service may be accepted and standardised and in this way choke the urge for continued improvement. It is doubtful whether there can be any wholly satisfactory compromise. It may be right for a limited period to accept the existing order of things—that is, quality in a small area—in the hope that its success will prompt others to proceed along similar lines. On the whole, the balance is in favour of quality, especially in a primary demonstration centre. It must be admitted sadly however, that a number of countries, even in Europe, have gleefully accepted a demonstration centre provided by some external Foundation and used it to show proudly to visitors, without any attempt on their own initiative to extend its benefits to other areas. These 'show-places' have only one advantage—that they can readily be turned into training centres and in this way at least serve the larger community. The remaining risk—voluntary bodies please note—is that the original centre in a country may be so elaborate and perfect that it arouses feelings of envy rather than a desire to extend and improve. The exhibition ought to be within the capacity of the receiving country, not merely in cost, but also in tradition. Perhaps the wisest policy is to make use of the first centre mainly as a demonstration area, recognised as such, and with just sufficient patients to serve this purpose. Overcrowding can do nothing but harm. The next step is to select suitable local candidates for training, with special reference to the choice of a site for the next centre. A second stage, which has been adopted with at least temporary success in a number of countries, is to use the central clinic as a service station for mobile teams. This procedure has at least this value—that it provides the teams with a focal point for reporting on their problems and successes, and it enables them to check and improve their equipment. In addition, this arrangement offers an opportunity for evaluation of the services, and particularly the effectiveness of the mobile units, for it should be clear that the mobile system is at best a temporary arrangement—the existing order of things pending the right solution: an advance post awaiting consolidation.

To sum up: great stress should be laid on the value of securing keen, understanding co-operation on a voluntary basis with the people on the spot. It is their goodwill and active support that will in the end determine the success or failure of a programme and the progress of community development. As a project develops and expands it is essential that it should incorporate plans for teaching, to raise standards through refresher courses for those who are already active, and to do everything possible to recruit auxiliary workers who show promise. Plans of this kind are determined at every stage by the operation of a team of highly trained workers in the health field who take responsibility for initiating and carrying through the programme and of assessing its progress. Leadership is indispensable, especially in the early stages. Introduced in this way, it matters little whether it starts as a mass campaign against disease, as a maternal and child health project, or as a plan to take over an existing scheme. Real progress comes from joint action between the state and the local community.

School Health

The subject of school health is in many ways more precise than the other personal health services. The main reason for this is that it came up at the beginning of this century as a service for a well-defined age group. The child at school was recognised as a convenient subject for study and medical care because many of the statistical facts are known, such as the name and address, the date of birth, attendance at school, the teacher's assessment of ability, and so on. From a statistical point of view the school child is a member of a 'captive population'. The fact that school health was not seriously examined until the early years of the present century is perhaps a matter of surprise, and still more that there was not a remarkable amount of voluntary effort to tackle the problem before the official schemes were adopted, under the Education Act. There are, however, reasons for this. The first is that compulsory school education was not made universal until a comparatively late date—the English Education Act being passed in 1871. In consequence, there had been very little time to put a system into action before doubts about physical fitness began to arise in the country generally. The first important step was in 1902, when a Scottish Royal Commission was appointed to enquire into the opportunities for physical training available in educational institutions, and to suggest means of making it conduce to the welfare of pupils. This Commission made some valuable recommendations, but I shall only quote their essential conclusion, which runs as follows:

The defects to which we have alluded in connection with the medical data now available points to a very serious defect in our school organisation, to which we desire to call special attention. This consists in the absence of any general or adequate system of medical inspection. Such a system is urgently demanded, mainly for remedial objectives, but also to make available information of the highest value, both for ascertaining the facts of national physique and the means that may be adopted for its improvement or for retarding such degeneration as may be in progress.

The Commission went on to point out that it was impossible to go beyond mere guesswork save by study and continuous collection of facts. The only way of getting these was by weighing and measuring and carefully estimating the condition of children and their status as to health. The Commission wisely pointed to the fact that the school period was the only age at which comprehensive information could be obtained, but this was not all: there were no uniform rules about the granting of medical certificates for illness, or the detecting and checking of infectious diseases. Only skilled medical examination could detect faults in sight or hearing or mental development, or physical weakness or poor nutrition. The Commission were convinced that defects in health and physique could be mitigated, if not removed, by timely attention. They pressed the importance of health education, which must be taught early if it is to become a matter of practice.

The wise and humble comments of this Report are just as necessary today as they were sixty years ago—especially the need to remember the little simple things about the nurture of children. Those who decry the school health service should bear in mind that the greatest proportion of the advances in children's health during the past half a century has been due not to striking modern remedies but to social education.

When children reach the middle school years, from about eight onwards, it is about then that boys begin to form groups of their own accord for games and other activities. Girls are more inclined to create individual friendships, and in any case their interests diverge a good deal. Groups of this kind deserve every encouragement, because they create an alternative interest to school work, and because they prevent loneliness and idling. In this respect, however, there is always a selection of 'unclubbable' boys and wretched, un-idea'd girls. They are the ones who are most prone to range around and get into mischief. In some cases, want of interest in organised groups is primarily due to apathetic parents, who do not realise that children who fail to join in group solidarity at this age are unlikely to do so later on. It is the general experience that teen-agers cannot be persuaded to join clubs and movements at fifteen or later unless they have had previous experience of the simpler forms of community life in Scout groups, Church and other voluntary activities.

SELECTIVE MEDICAL INSPECTION

From the point of view of international progress, it might be desirable to have regard for recent modifications in the system of school medical inspection. The main reason for this is that the proposals which have been brought forward in a considerable number of areas since Dorothy Nyswander made her original report for the Commonwealth Fund in 1942 have certain advantages, especially where shortage of medical staff is a serious consideration.

The Chief Medical Office of the Ministry of Education commented on a number of these experiments in 1958, and since then many authorities have set up a plan for what is known now as the selective method of school medical inspection. A good example of this was reported by Lionel Bacon as a result of an experiment in Hampshire.

The essential features of this system are that the older routine inspection of children in the intermediate period between entry and leaving has been greatly modified. The entrants' inspection has been retained and is regarded as especially important because it is now the only school medical inspection which *every* child receives. The leavers' inspection has been retained but it is rather an interview at which the child's health is briefly reviewed from previous reports and enquiries are made about his proposed occupation, especially in relation to any disability which he may have. The leaver is asked about any worries that he may have concerning his own health, and he is medically examined only if there seems to be a special need. Throughout the whole of the rest of a child's school life he is liable to be *selected* for medical inspection. To a large extent this is only an extension of the previous system of providing for 'specials' to be brought forward by the head teacher, the parents or the nurse at any medical inspection. The difference, however, is that under the older system there was no organised search for children who ought to be examined, and the number of 'specials' was therefore relatively small and limited. The new procedure provides for a 'selection visit' by the medical officer each term to decide which of the children shall be medically examined. It is basically an interview with the head teacher by appointment. The essential procedure consists of:

1. A questionnaire to be completed by all parents.
2. Information provided by the head teacher.
3. Information provided by the school nurse.
4. Direct observation of the children at physical education or at play by the school medical officer.

The questionnaire alone may give sufficient grounds for selection, as frequently it indicates that the child has something the matter with him, and in this case the medical officer makes his decision after discussion with the nurse and the head teacher. The medical officer now conducts a rapid review, with the head of the school, of all the children to whom the questionnaires relate, even if the child has apparently a clean bill of health, and in this way the sieve is made finer.

The head teacher's contribution has proved to be of great value, but of course in large schools this contribution depends upon consultation with the children's own class teachers also. Not infrequently the head teacher invites the medical officer to meet the class teachers, but that is at his own discretion. The value of the school nurse's contribution depends largely on her knowledge of the homes and parents of the children. This is specially useful in helping the medical officer to interpret the questionnaire, and it maintains the nurse's interest in the whole procedure and probably helps in her own visits to the homes.

The fourth item of the selection visit—direct observation of the children—has not been so useful as was hoped. Its value lies in a few details only: *e.g.*, the opportunity to observe footwear, and posture, and faults of the orthopaedic kind. It also has the

secondary advantage, which is a very real one, of allowing the
school medical officer to enter the classrooms and see the
children as a group.

In looking back on the planning of this scheme, and reviewing
the first two years of its working, Dr. Bacon notes that one
thing stands out clearly: they set out to devise an improved
defect-finding procedure and they found that they had obtained
an opportunity for greatly improved doctor/teacher relationships. There were of course difficulties at the start, and there
remained some in the detailed organisation of the scheme,
but there was a feeling that the medical officer on his side had
learned more about the difficulties that his advice in the case of
children with defects might entail for the school staff.

The results of the inspection itself were more difficult to
assess, and it would require a much longer period of study to
know whether this type of examination was more or less complete than those under the old system. It was almost certain,
however, that the selection term by term would show at an
earlier period any defect which had newly arisen, especially
orthopaedic defects such as round backs and flat feet, and there
was some reason to believe that the new system led to a greater
knowledge of psychological defects in school children, which
could be discussed in detail with the teaching staff. The number
of psychological difficulties reported has increased under this
system, but this may indicate no more than a more careful
assessment of possibly transient emotional troubles.

A system of this kind, speaking more generally, is likely to be
more elastic in countries which have difficulties in staffing and
in providing skilled medical attention. The provision of nurses
instead of doctors may be all that is possible in many areas, but
that at any rate is more satisfactory than routine inspections
which would require definite medical qualifications. The
advantage is that the nurses are more readily able to select
from their own experience children who appear to require
attention, and these could be sorted out according to the
amount of care available.

My own experience of the school medical service covers quite
a long period from 1919 to 1937, and a considerable variety of
areas including a compact county borough and three county
councils. In addition, I was able to increase my experience

through studies in a number of European countries and also in the United States.

The relationship between the school health officer and the local general practitioner is all-important. I have seen a considerable variety of usage—from the doctor who works part-time in the school medical service in the midst of a busy general practice to the whole-time officer of the local authority. My own feeling is that school medical inspection belongs essentially to the education programme, and should therefore be carried out by an officer of the local authority. It is of course possible, and in some cases preferable, that the general practitioner should be responsible for the duties of school medical inspection to the local authority, but in practice there are a number of objections to this. The school medical officer is not concerned with clinical work as such, but rather with the broader issues of health and deviations resulting from prolonged sickness of defects. The general practitioner is in most cases content to receive reports from the school health service and to deal with the patient and his family as a personal matter. This is quite different from ante-natal care and obstetric work generally, where the practitioner is dealing clinically with an individual and must in the nature of things be responsible for all matters concerning pregnancy and the health and future care of the young child. In that case there is no question of the health department coming in, except in relation to group teaching of expectant mothers, and mothers in the early period of their family life.

The same answer applies to the care of the pre-school child. The doctor in charge of the family should be primarily responsible for this duty. It is only when questions arise about mental or physical defect, or other disabilities of long duration, that the school medical service has a duty and a special value. One characteristic illustration of special care lies in the physically defective, because the care of a child with this kind of disability, whatever the cause, is a special concern of the educational service. Moreover, while the family doctor has obviously a keen interest and responsibility for the child as requiring medical care, there comes a time when the weight of importance swings to the educational side, and the care of the defective child as a member of the community, perhaps requiring edu-

D

cation in a special school, or apparatus which is beyond the capacity of the parents to supply and keep in order, or more or less continued supervision by the public health nurse. The same, with modifications, applies to the child who is suffering from mental disorder or requiring guidance on account of certain difficulties in relation to school work and taking his part in community life.

The same considerations apply, although for a different reason, to certain special examinations which are more or less routinely carried out by the educational service and which save a good deal of public money and parental anxiety. This applies particularly to dental care and to defects of the eyes and ears. In most areas it is found that specially appointed educational medical officers save the general practitioner an enormous amount of time and anxiety by undertaking at least the preliminary stages of such examinations. If, of course, a serious condition of the eyes or ears supervenes, the family doctor would be responsible for advising the parents, and any further help needed could be obtained by means of specialists.

The next point which has an overwhelming importance in the school medical service is the collaboration between the school medical officer and the teaching service. One of the factors which contributes greatly to the benefit of the child is co-ordination between the teaching and the medical profession, and this can be carried out satisfactorily only in the community service provided by the schools themselves. There is an additional point in the close relationship between teaching and school medicine: that the state of the school as a whole from the point of view of structure and safety (e.g. from infectious disease) can be supervised as a routine by collaboration between teachers and medical officers. The same kind of co-operation applies to school nurses and voluntary workers.

The parents of the children are in a special category. In most systems, of course, their consent is required to the actual examination, and in some countries this consent is limited by all kinds of restrictions. Active interest is best shown by the presence of the parent at the school medical examination, so that any question relating to the health and welfare of the child can be discussed between the school medical officer and the parent and, if desirable, the head teacher.

A final matter of importance is a good relationship between parent, doctor and nurse. Some authorities have separated the care of the pre-school child wholly from the school medical service. Others have felt that it adds interest to school medical work for doctor and nurse to follow the same course throughout the child's life until he leaves school. Whatever plan is adopted, there should be opportunities for the nurse to visit the parents in their homes. This is particularly important in the follow-up of defective children, but it is also valuable in educational work. Looking to the future, it seems probable that the main division in medical care will lie between the general practitioner, who will take increasing responsibility for obstetrical work and ante-natal services on the one hand and for the young child before school age on the other, and the school medical service, which will maintain supervision over the whole of school life as part of the educational system of the country.

Chapter 4

SOCIAL DIAGNOSIS

In recent years, as we have seen, multitudes of people, both professional and lay, have been ramming home to us the importance of the 'social factor' in health and sickness. The most progressive of our clinical colleagues, looking at the problem from their own way of thinking, have referred to the *social factor* in the study of disease in such a way that disease is considered not in isolation but against the background of home and family, work and play. This important subject, under the title of *social pathology*, was finely developed by Ryle in his book *Changing Disciplines*[1]. It has since been imitated by many with less understanding. In Ryle's concept of social pathology the clinician would aim at letting the medical student see the pattern of disease woven into the background of home, family, work and other basic material. In this concept the position of the medical social worker is pivotal and the social worker as a member of the team to teach undergraduate students is indispensable. The use of the social worker in this capacity was first developed by Richard Cabot of Boston in the year 1906, and it has gradually spread through many clinical schools in the United States, in this country and elsewhere. The developments in the United States have been ably described by one of Cabot's early pupils, Ida Cannon, in her book 'On the social frontier of medicine—pioneering in medical social science'. This concept of social pathology is valuable, especially in the hospital service, but it has the disadvantage that it begins with manifest disease.

I have referred to social pathology today, only to distinguish it from social diagnosis which is much more concerned with prevention, and comes within the scope of the medical officer of health and the health visitor even more than the medical social worker who is based on the hospital. To put the matter very briefly, social diagnosis has the following characteristics:—

1. It is based primarily on the home and not on the hospital.
2. It is concerned in the first instance with health and its

maintenance and not with sickness and its cure. The visiting of expectant and nursing mothers, of infants, young children and school children, are examples of the application of social diagnosis.

3. Social diagnosis looks to the family as a whole rather than to an individual member; as an illustration of this one may cite a family in which one member has tuberculosis. Social diagnosis extends beyond the individual patient to the reaction of tuberculosis on the other members and the general relationship of the patient to his family.

4. It is not mainly concerned with medical diagnosis (which is usually fully known) but with any social problem which may lie behind the medical problem and will be essential for guidance, education and comfort.

5. Social diagnosis is essentially practical and realistic; concerned with adjustment to life as it is, and not with remote policies whether social or political. It is concerned, for example, with a housing problem, or with the difficulties concerning a defective who cannot be admitted to an institution.

Now we have to consider how this affects the staff of a health service, such as the medical officer of health or a health visitor. I think we can say at once that it fits into their immediate duties, and I shall include among the duties in this respect four essential items:—

1. To advise on health and its maintenance in the health centre or clinic, the home and the work place. It is his duty to advise people in the group, in the family or as individuals.

2. To advise on the prevention of sickness at the earliest possible stage of deviation from normal health. The object of this is to provide a check against more serious illness and protect others from the risk of infection.

3. To protect the community when danger threatens. The medical officer of health is not concerned with the niceties of infectious disease in diagnosis. His duty is to err on the side of safety and the price of safety is eternal vigilance. The medical officer of health and his staff must therefore make a constant study of the pattern of sickness in the community and this applies to all sickness whether it is manifestly epidemic or otherwise.

4. To organise a *service* of health in his local community and

with the confidence and support of the local authority, that is the elected representatives of the people. Local government has no doubt many faults. We hear stories of corruption, of stupidity and of niggardly finance. Some of these are no doubt true but what is the alternative? (Winifred Holtby: South Riding).

But when I came to consider local government, I began to see how it was in essence the first-line defence thrown up by the community against our common enemies—poverty, sickness, ignorance, isolation, mental derangement and social maladjustment. The battle is not faultlessly conducted, nor are the motives of those who take part in it *all* righteous or disinterested. But the war is, I believe, worth fighting, and this corporate action is at least based upon recognition of one fundamental truth about human nature—we are not only single individuals, each face to face with eternity and our separate spirits; we are members one of another.

Now we come to the practical side of social diagnosis. Suppose, for the sake of illustration, that a member of a family under your charge as a health officer requires public medical care; it might be because of some long-term illness, such as poliomyelitis or tuberculosis and for convenience we shall speak of the person who is the focus of your visit to the home as 'the patient'. The first duty of the health officer is to collect the social *evidence* about the patient and his family; that is the relevant facts about his personal and family history and the environment as actually seen on the visit. These two, when taken together, give a picture of your patient in relation to the problem to be studied; illness, maladjustment, bad housing, the problems raised by the arrival of a new baby, the difficulties to be faced with a mentally defective child and so on. In obtaining social evidence you have much greater scope than if you were dealing with legal evidence because you are free to handle indirect information—what is sometimes called hearsay evidence— which you cannot do in a court of law, and to draw inferences from all kinds of impressions. There is an obvious danger in accepting indirect evidence where strict proof is required, as in a criminal case, but it is extremely useful when your understanding of the situation depends NOT so much on the facts as on your interpretation of what you see and hear. Some facts are direct and simple and can be noted down without difficulty, e.g. the number of rooms in a house, the number of people and their ages and sex. The

supreme risk, when you are making a social diagnosis, is not
the misuse of evidence but the danger of asking leading questions, that is questions which suggest the answer that you want.
The classical example of a leading question is 'When did you
stop beating your wife?' A more simple one, and possibly more
appropriate for the present day is 'When did you last give the
baby cod liver oil?' The same applies to questions clothed with a
judgment—'Surely you did not use that dirty rag?' Or 'Has not
that jam been lying on the table cloth for weeks?'—so putting
your feelings in front of the quest for the truth. Nothing is more
likely to destroy mutual understanding.

Now we come to the process of questioning. The first communication which probably comes from the office to the home
is important; not very long ago I read this letter when I was
visiting a house: 'Dear Madam, I am instructed to visit your
dwelling on Monday, 15th October at 2.30 p.m. Kindly
arrange to make yourself available at that time.' So please
write a human and personal note; say who you are and what
you do. Tell the people that you hope your visit will be convenient and give them an opportunity to change the time. Of
course it is not always possible or desirable to write in advance.
When I was doing my earlier housing visits in the Midlands I
was looking for slum property. It was therefore impossible to
write beforehand as I did not know the houses, let alone the
families, that I wanted to see; so I used to turn up early in the
morning at a town or village armed with a large scale map. I
made a quick walk round noting on the map property which was
obviously deteriorating or decayed. Having done that I went
back to the car and strengthened myself with a cup of coffee
from a thermos flask and sallied forth once more at about 9.30
a.m. when I was sure the children would have gone to school.
After some experience of trial and error I found a very simple
technique which worked in almost every case. I called at each
house in turn and told the housewife who I was and why I was
there and said that I was interested in looking at houses, especially those that needed repair, and then said quickly 'but, of
course, it may not be convenient for you to show me round just
now, although I don't expect you to be tidy at this time of the
morning.' In approximately half the cases I was invited in
immediately with a friendly apology for untidiness. In the

other half there was a moment's hesitation and I immediately said 'How would it do if I called in the afternoon?' That accounted for practically the whole of the remainder. I only remember five instances out of five thousand where I was refused admission and in only two I was treated with a show of violence. One of the women chased me down the garden with a broom on a wet morning and I escaped through a hedge.

Interviews about housing, however, are relatively easy because you are looking at objective things. When you are going to see a patient, member of a family, it is much more difficult because success or failure may well depend on your first approach and determine the whole of your subsequent relations with the family. On the whole it is easier for a medical social worker than for other types of visitor such as those who are enquiring about a mentally defective child or someone who is on probation. On the medical side people are generally more friendly because they like to talk about their ailments and their children; in fact their ailments become their children. The main job in the first visit is to gain the confidence of the family as a foundation for building up further interviews. The objects of the first interview are therefore:—

1. Give a fair hearing. It is more blessed to listen than to talk.

2. To establish a sympathetic understanding so that your patient will turn to you again in time of difficulty.

3. Try to get your information tactfully where you are asking questions and where there is any difficulty stop and look for your clues from other sources.

4. Get their consent to further enquiries.

5. Remember that your first visit has a great therapeutic value if it is rightly conducted. You give to the family a sense of your interest and sympathy. Keep your criticism until you know them better.

I should like to elaborate on one or two of these points. First the fair hearing. The method of your approach is designed because you have to overcome the patient's natural reserve and your own. This is not an easy matter. It does not help to slobber all over them. Begin with general questions; for example about the patient's comfort; things on which you will get a ready reply without seeming to probe and then you can make an easy move to the history of the patient's illness or trouble, whatever the matter may be. Avoid above all, at this stage, the notebook and the form and the spate of questions. Later when you gain the patient's confidence you may be quite frank and ask permission to confirm some of the points made by taking notes. It is quite easy to say 'I am sure you would want me to make a note of some of these things so that later on I do not ask the same thing over again'. Do not waste time by pushing stubbornly at questions which are avoided in the first instance. (That rule applies equally to examiners in public health). It is better to follow indirect clues, the information that other people can give you, than to become petulant about what is grudgingly revealed. Next, in dealing with sick and elderly people a frequent change of subject avoids fatigue. If you have only patience enough to give people time their answers will always be more revealing and helpful than if you go forward hastily with a thorough cross-examination.

It is of the greatest importance to promote understanding and you may have to forgo information for the sake of getting a better understanding, at least in the first instance. There is a tremendous value in allowing your witness to tell his own story and you should avoid interruptions or even attempts to fill in the gaps in a story when the patient hesitates.

In following up clues do not bypass the patient unless
(a) you were actually requested by him to get the information from some other source, or the patient readily consents to your request;
(b) that it is absolutely necessary in order to establish a diagnosis. When you have to bypass the patient try to seek the most disinterested opinions, such as the Family Welfare Association, the teacher in the case of a school child, medical or nursing opinion in the case of a sick person.

The therapeutic value of social diagnosis will be greatly enhanced if you remember a few simple points:—do not ask questions *in vacuo*; have a purpose and if your first plan fails be ready to adopt a new plan—not chaos. Some prefer a fixed order of procedure and certainly that is the best method for beginners; learn the main questions by heart and stick to a recognisable order. More experienced questioners can use any method they like and put the questions back into the right order when they are reviewing the case. This gives a better sense of conversation and informality but it is much more difficult.

Now let me try to sum up the rules of the game:—

1. Do not start with an abrupt question which feels like a cold hand on a hot abdomen.

2. Be cautious with your notebook. You are not there as a member of the police force or a detective.

3. When a direct question is necessary explain the reason first, otherwise your question will often sound rude and abrupt, especially when you are perhaps opening up an unhappy subject like the loss of a child.

4. Frame your questions so as to bring out the truth and not your own opinions.

5. With a sick or a difficult person do not ask what you can just as well obtain elsewhere, e.g., the ordinary facts about a patient's name, age and so on.

6. Do not ask useless questions just because you cannot think of anything to say. Change the subject.

7. Avoid the great temptation of making promises or giving advice prematurely. This brings only discredit on you and the authority which you serve. There is always a risk about this because it is the easiest way to impress a patient or to get information from a reluctant dragon; for example in a housing investigation avoid talking about the prospects of a new house.

8. Weigh your evidence afterwards when you are making a final note so as to arrive at the true interpretation of the problem, its cause, its remedy, and the outlook in terms of social progress.

We come, as in chess, to what is called the end game. On closing the interview ask yourself:—

1. Has all the really essential information been obtained?

2. Is there any half-hidden resentment which may damage the future relations?

3. End if you can on a hopeful note, without referring to funerals, or test matches, or the state of China or Berlin.

And lastly,

4. Remember the student's job is to study and get information, not to engage in propaganda, criticism, or condemnation. You may say what you like about the weather.

REFERENCES

[1]RYLE, J. A. (1948): *Changing Discipline,* Oxford University Press.

Chapter 5

TEACHING AND PRACTICE
OF PUBLIC HEALTH

The attitude of the medical profession to the public health officer has been discussed and illustrated in many countries, notably the United States and the United Kingdom. The subject is of special interest at the present time, when new experiments in the pattern of medical practice are being made. One might cite Canada, Chile and the U.S.S.R. as obvious examples; but in many other countries, especially those which have recently acquired independence, as in Africa, there is evidence of changing patterns and directions. It must be admitted that in some cases these changes are being adopted by Government decree and the teaching centres and medical profession—if indeed they have any voice in the matter—are undertaking a rearguard action. One probable reason for this is that the profession has a strong tradition of individualism, whereas public authorities are more concerned with communities.

Sir John Charles, in his final report as Chief Medical Officer of the Ministry of Health, made an excellent summary of the functions of the Medical Officer of Health today. Any assumption, he said, that the function of the health officer is likely to diminish in scope and value is based on an unimaginative approach to the realities of the present situation and is something else than a compliment to those men of vision in the past whose labours have contributed so much to the improvement in national health within a lifetime. Not only have these enhanced standards to be maintained, but still further advances to deal with existing ill-health demand much more thought, study and attention.

The health officer, Sir John continues, who should increasingly regard himself as a community physician, occupies a special place of vantage. As the leader of a public health team he is something more than a departmental organiser; indeed, in the larger areas much of the day to day procedure is a function of his senior medical and administrative staff. With his background of training and experience in general and in social medicine, it is the medical officer of health's responsibility to maintain a strategical survey of the business of his department. Avoiding undue preoccupation with details, which should more properly be left to others, he should ensure that he is in effect keeping a careful watch on the course which his department as a whole is following, and on the relationships which are being maintained between the various members of his staff. It is essential, therefore, that there should be frequent staff conferences and discussions within his department, and between the department and the various cognate services such as engineering, education, public assistance and architecture. The environmental, the personal, the welfare and the mental health services to which Sir John Charles refers, are now integral parts of one community health service.

These community functions were little understood in the United Kingdom until the present century was well advanced, and indeed the current organisation of public health services would have met with astonishment and incredulity in the health officers of the previous age, that is, before the first world war. At that time public health as a discipline was related to the German concept and its teaching throughout Europe was generally associated with the sciences, such as bacteriology and tropical diseases which have made such enormous advances towards the close of the nineteenth and in the first decade of the twentieth century.

Some public health officers in the United Kingdom felt that the organisation which they served had reached its zenith during the second world war and was then going into a decline. The reasons for this suspicion were not founded mainly on the transfer of hospitals to the Minister of Health under the National Health Service, or on similar adjustments in relation to tuberculosis, venereal diseases, and the like, although these revolutionary changes swept away many of the health officer's functions, especially in the county boroughs. The deeper causes for disquiet in the health services depended on principles determining the trends of present day legislation, its outlook and its limitations. A wise medical officer of health in his annual report for the year 1901 wrote as follows:

May I be allowed to say that the science of Public Health has both an objective and an ethical side. The former is represented by the routine work of a Sanitary Department—nuisances, drainage, infection, and their respective control. The ethical side is of infinitely greater importance, for it is more lasting in its effects, aiming as it does at the production of a cleaner, purer, and richer social life. The science of public health has in fact been said truly to be in essence the application of scientific medicine to present social circumstances. Local authorities, by the organisation of measures for the improvement of the environment of the individual must eventually succeed in raising the standard of civilized life. *

The National Health Service Act of 1946 was concerned primarily with the medical and nursing care of the sick. The use of the term 'health' in the Act carried no conviction to the health officer, because the problems which it dealt with were vague and ill-defined in comparison with the Sections dealing with treatment. At best they related to the prevention of sickness in the individual, and bore little reference to the community as a whole. This is not a criticism of the Act as such, except in so far as its title is a misnomer and may be misleading to the public. The organisation for medical care had been in a state of confusion, and the Statute provided admirably for the better distribution of services, including specialist and laboratory facilities. Moreover, as we have seen, it brought back into the fold of general medicine the clinical care of a number of conditions which for one reason and another had strayed into the realm of the public health services. In fact, it strengthened the very point which Ryle made:

Hitherto, our science, like our practice, has evolved along individualist lines. Whatever the several countries may do with regard to the modification of their systems of practice and of service, it seems to me that the scientific study of health and disease in man—the most complex of all social animals—must henceforward concern itself to an ever-increasing degree with the interactions and correlations of disease and health with changing social circumstance. Socially, industrially, politically, we are creating a new age. With it, inevitably, we alter the whole character and distribution of diseases and set ourselves new problems for solution in the fields of medical science, practice and administration.[1]

* Dr. Meredith Young of Stockport, Annual Report, 1901.

Well devised arrangements were made in the Act for broadening the scope of consultant services, with the object of making available to every person at the moment of need unrestricted access to the best medical care that modern science can provide. The general practitioner service was extended to cover the entire population and a real attempt was made to distribute doctors according to the needs of patients rather than on the basis of eligibility of practice. In other words, the new Act aimed at providing a comprehensive system of medical care for the whole population free of cost at time of need. From the point of view of preventive medicine this was a notable advance, but most unhappily it ignored two vital factors which were closely interrelated. The first of these was the stimulation of general practice to take part in the great team work of the new service, and the second was to link the hospital and specialist services with general practice and with public health. Substantial improvements have been made from within in relation to general practice, mainly through the influence of the College of General Practitioners, which was founded in 1952. Since that time, owing to the vision of its promoters, the whole concept of general practice has progressively widened its boundaries—by the stimulation of group research and by fruitful co-operation with the health services.

On the other hand, the proposals for dealing with the health services left many problems unsettled. It is hardly open to question that the great structure already built by the local authorities, including maternity and child welfare, the school medical and dental services, health visiting, the human aspects of housing, and all the personal services rendered by the health officer and his staff, have contributed in the last half century to the steady improvement in the health of the community. This is clearly represented in the vital statistics of Britain and many other countries. In this connection, however, those who framed the National Health Service appeared to give less attention, and even to overlook, two points. The first is that the prevention of sickness and the promotion of health are community services as well as individual. There is a parallel in the education service: it is quite possible to educate a child in his own home, but no-one but a fanatic would suggest that the education of every child should be undertaken in his family circle. If that were possible it would still be wrong in principle, because there is an intrinsic value in teaching children as a community—as members of one another. In this way they learn how to give and take, how to live together as citizens, and how to work and play in harmony. At the present time a similar problem has become urgent in relation to the practice of medicine. While we lay a just emphasis on the individual and family responsibility, we cannot afford to neglect the community aspects, that is the conscious and skilled teaching of health.

The second point is that, contrary to the views expressed by many at the present time, the health officer is not concerned merely with an impersonal phenomenon called the community. He must be continuously in touch with persons, both in their individual capacities and as members of families. In point of fact the health officer has been a practitioner of what is now called social medicine for several generations. Much of his teaching is rightly directed to people in groups, such as clinics for expectant mothers, infant welfare centres, and schools; for that is the essence of teaching methods in which he is a trained practitioner. To take a single example: housing, for the health officer, should not be merely a question of considering whether a dwelling is fit or unfit for habitation by some rule of thumb standard, or by the application of local by-laws. It involves for every medical officer of health a careful consideration of the house as a home, its fitness in relation to the needs of the particular family that occupies the house. The average general practitioner is called to visit a house when a member of the family is sick. It is essential that he should become, in co-operation with the health service, not merely a medical attendant to the sick person, but also a health adviser to the families under his care. At the same time this aspect of medicine may be overstressed, especially by those who regard the health officer of today as interested mainly in such subjects as maternal and child care, the health of the aged, and many other elements of public health which are predominantly social in character. There is a risk that the medical officers of health themselves may be weaned away from their functions and duties and forget that, in spite of the great enlargement of the field of their endeavour, the prime function of the health officer is today unchanged in scope and in responsibility. The English General

Board of Health on 20 December 1855 issued the following instructions, and many of these are just as valid today as they were over a century ago:

The officer of health is appointed in order that through him the local sanitary authority may be duly informed of such influences as are acting against the healthiness of the population of his district, and of such steps as medical science can advise for their removal; secondly, to execute such special functions as may devolve upon him by the statute under which he is appointed; and thirdly, to contribute to that general stock of knowledge with regard to the sanitary condition of the people and to the preventible causes of sickness and mortality which, when collected, methodized, and reported to Parliament by the General Board of Health, may guide the Legislature in the extension and amendment of sanitary law.

The duties of the officer of health will be to the following effect:—

1. He will make himself familiar with the natural and acquired features of the place, with the social and previous sanitary state of its population, and with all its existing provisions for health—namely, with the levels, inclinations, soils, wells, and watersprings of the district; with its meteorological peculiarities; with the distribution of its buildings and open spaces, paved or unpaved, of its burial-grounds and lay-stalls; with the plan of its drains, sewers, and water supply; with the nature of its manufacturing and other industrial establishments; with the house accommodation of the poorer classes, and their opportunities for bathing and washing; with the arrangements for burial of the dead, and with the regulations in force for lodginghouses and slaughtering-places, for the cleansing of public ways and markets, and for the removal of domestic refuse.

2. He will invite communications relating to the sanitary wants of the district from the resident clergy, the medical practitioners, registrars, relieving officers, and other persons or societies engaged in the visitation of the poor.

3. He will take the best means in his power to become acquainted from week to week, and in times of severe disease from day to day, with the deaths and sicknesses in his district; and he will enquire to what extent they have depended on removeable causes.

4. With the assistance of such subordinate officers as the local board may empower him to direct and superintend, he will watch his district, taking care to bring its several parts under examination

as often as their sanitary circumstances shall require, and especially observing those places which have previously given occasion of complaint, or been subject to sickness. He will enquire as to the cleanly, wholesome, and weatherproof condition of houses; as to their due ventilation and not overcrowded condition; as to the efficiency of their drainage and water supply; and as to the absence of dampness and offensive effluvia in and about them. He will examine from time to time the drinking waters of the place, and will observe whether provisions are offered for sale in any damaged or adulterated state that is hurtful or illegal. He will occasionally visit all burial-places, and see whether they give any ground for complaint, and he will habitually observe the slaughtering houses of the district and other industrial establishments which are liable to emit offensive (especially animal) effluvia.

It is remarkable how closely the Ministry of Health instruction follows the same lines three quarters of a century later:

The chief function of the Medical Officer of Health is to safeguard the health of the area for which he acts by such means as are at his disposal, and to advise his Authority how knowledge of public health and preventive medicine can be made available and utilised for the benefit of the community. He should endeavour to acquire an accurate knowledge of the influences, social, environmental and industrial, which may operate prejudicially, to health in the area, and of the agencies, official or unofficial, whose help can be invoked in amelioration of such influences. While he has special duties for the prevention of infectious diseases, all morbid conditions contributing to a high sickness rate or mortality in the area from these or other causes should be studied with a view to their prevention or control.[2]

What then are the future tasks of the Health Department? This question has been answered very ably by Dr. I. A. G. MacQueen:

The main future tasks of the health department are to improve emotional and social health; to preserve the health and well-being of veterans; to support and rehabilitate persons handicapped by physical, mental or social disability; to reduce non-infectious diseases; and to continue to eliminate environmental hazards. For these tasks we need knowledge of child psychology and social psychology; health education skills; discussion techniques and methods; physiology and disease processes; sociology; epidemiological techniques; hygiene and sanitation; and (since departments are large) staff management and administration.[3]

E

The term 'social Medicine' has become widely used, and different groups of workers, scientific and others, are making use of it. There is, in the first place, the austere presentation of the human comedy in which men and women are units which can be moved about according to certain statistical rules, and are then grouped to form significant relationships. We may learn much from these studies: indeed many of them form a framework on which new knowledge may be constructed. These form the basis of valuable research in social medicine. At the other extreme, we see artless and benevolent social work. This may be represented by social surveys of bewildering variety from strike ballots in the medical professional to solicitous enquiries about the heights of sinks and the pattern of gas rings. Social medicine, at best, rises to the level of skilled social survey, and at worst it is a political rather than a social weapon.

Between these extremes lies the level of social medicine— which boasts two soul-sides. The first is essentially clinical and personal. It brings the student sharply against the family as a social unit, and the patient as a member of that family. When I was a medical student we were taken round the wards by competent clinicians. We noted that a patient had oedema of the ankles and was breathless on exertion, but we did not picture that woman standing by a machine for hours on end, and then having to climb four flights of stairs in her tenement at night to attend to the home and the evening meal. We observed the crepitations in the man suffering from phthisis and (with luck) saw in the stained specimen of sputum the tubercle bacillus standing out, bright red against the misty blue background. But we did not see the darker background of the patient—the long struggle against hopeless odds to keep his family going, and the perilous state of that family when he had at last broken down.

The second is the community aspect of medicine, practised faithfully by the good general practitioner for generations, and more recently by the good medical officer of health, but insufficiently recognised by his masters, the public.

The first approach to social medicine came through sanitary reform—the attack on bad housing and shocking environmental conditions. Then came the great fusion at the end of the nineteenth century—the union of personal and environmental health; this has been properly called the 'Age of Personal Health'. Its aim is essentially educative and its patient is the community.

We may now return to the subject of Preventive Medicine in the broad sense. Even the briefest outline of the evolution of teaching in the subject would be incomplete without reference to the work of H. W. Rumsey, whose essays on State Medicine (1856) contributed so much to education and practice. His caustic observations on the failure of the Government to provide medical education must have given rise to some heart-searchings:

> To train and prepare youths for medical and sanitary employment is elsewhere to be one of the most serious responsibilities of Government. It is one which no nation has ever neglected without loss to the State and injury to the people. Yet it is one which English Governments and Parliaments have strenuously shunned, for it affects neither political influence nor party ascendency. A loud and importunate outcry for intervention must arise before they can be induced even to shift their own responsibilities, in this matter, upon medical corporations. But to take the initiative, and especially to found professorships in various branches of the healing and health-preserving arts, has been considered a kind of political Quixotism, of which no sober-minded English minister could possibly be guilty.

The scandals of hospital administration during the Crimean War had a powerful influence on the teaching of public health through the medium of Edmund Parkes, whose brilliant work in Army sanitation led to his appointment in 1860 as Professor of Military Hygiene in the first Army Medical School. Parkes was an able teacher as well as a practical hygienist, and his publication in 1864 of his famous 'Manual of Practical Hygiene', laid the foundations of the subject as a science which could be taught in the laboratory and in the field. In 1863, Parkes was appointed a Crown Member of the General Medical Council, a position in which he exerted great influence in promoting medical education and especially post-graduate teaching in public health.

Opinion was not all on one side, even among scientists. At the time when Acland was experimenting in field studies, Billroth,[4] in order to emphasise the value of the basic sciences, confessed that he was not interested in the struggle for public health. 'If

the whole of Social Medicine', he said, 'must needs be part of
the curriculum of the medical student, it must not take more
than two hours per semester, let us say, during the last two
semesters; otherwise it will surely be detrimental to his other
studies. This subject will never greatly interest the student, for
he will have his hands full in dealing with the diseases of the
individual, and will take as little interest in the community
welfare as he has in practical politics and diplomacy.'

This opinion represented the extreme German view of teaching in public health, and W. H. Welch carried it with him to
Baltimore, when he became Professor of Pathology in 1884 at
Johns Hopkins. Insistence at that time on a thorough grounding
in the basic sciences was of extreme value in raising the standards of medical education in America. Many years later, when
Welch resigned his University chair and set himself, at the age
of sixty-six, to organise the new School of Hygiene, he rightly
regarded the School as an institute for research; but at the
same time he showed the breadth of his vision and statesmanship by adding:

> I am trying to stress the humanistic aspect of Medicine because
> in the past the whole emphasis was, in my case, and I think the
> times demanded that emphasis, upon the purely scientific side.

In these words Welch raised the standard for a revolution in
teaching and practice. At that time specialisation in public
health was a new concept in America, and the ground was clear
for building.

It has often been pointed out that there is a great gap between
the establishment of scientific knowledge and its application to
human needs. This time-lag is partly due to economic causes,
partly to lack of administrative machinery, and perhaps in part
to insufficient diffusion of knowledge to the executive officer.
A gap of the same kind occurs between the recognition of the
needs of a service, and the fulfilment of these needs through
adaptation of teaching methods. The necessary changes are
often expensive and the administrative machine grinds slowly;
they may involve persons who have to alter routine methods or
even abandon cherished subjects of instruction.

It is essential that a course of teaching in such a subject as
preventive medicine should be elastic and capable of ready
adaptation to changing needs. We are living in a revolution and,

as Julian Huxley said in a recent work, we should learn 'to think in terms of direction and rate of change instead of goals or blueprints or defined systems, however ideal.'[5]

It is in these terms that we should examine the requirements of public health teaching and practice. The first question to be asked is quite simple: 'What are the needs of the medical officer of health today?' It is clear that this question should be repeated at reasonable intervals if we are to think in terms of direction and rate of change. In my view the primary aim of a School or University Department of Hygiene is to make good general practitioners in health; to send forth keen, competent men and women, with a high sense of their calling and a scientific outlook. It is easy to say these brave words, but difficult to translate them into an organised teaching course. There are, however, certain principles for our guidance:

1. No School or University can create a scientific outlook in its students unless it is actively engaged in research in the basic sciences. By this I mean science for the advancement of knowledge irrespective of 'practical' considerations.

2. The Department should direct the application of scientific work to the problems of public health, e.g., through surveys, routine laboratory investigations, statistical and epidemiological studies, and field experiment.

3. The Department should be directly associated with current health administration, including housing and sanitation, institutions and hospitals, and the everyday duties of the practising medical officer of health.

4. The Department should co-ordinate the postgraduate course in Public Health by direct teaching of the principles of social or community medicine, in order to weld the course of training into a coherent whole. It is the duty of the professor of preventive medicine to see that the course is complete, sound in structure, balanced in emphasis, and sufficient as a framework for the building of experience.

I wish to turn now to the special functions of a 'School of Hygiene'. The earliest examples of schools designed as colleges of preventive medicine are the School of Hygiene and Public Health at Johns Hopkins University, the University of Toronto School of Hygiene, and the London School of Hygiene and Tropical Medicine. These three institutions drew much of their inspiration from a report prepared in 1915 by Dr. W. H. Welch and Mr. Wickliffe Rose and presented to the General Education Board of the Rockefeller Foundation, and their success could not have been achieved without the consistent and generous support of the Foundation. The germinal ideas of the Johns Hopkins School serve as a fine illustration of my theme. The essential proposals were that the school should give weight both to the scientific aspects of hygiene and to the practical task of preparing candidates for public health positions. It was emphasised that the school should be independent of the medical school but closely related to it— this relation to be secured by the use of clinical facilities and general access to the teaching hospital, so far as was necessary for the postgraduate student in public health and the needs of the research work. The scope of training was not to obscure the conception of hygiene as a science and art which is much broader than its applications to public health administration. 'A main function of the school should be the development of the spirit of investigation and the advancement of knowledge.'

The Welch-Rose Report also laid great stress on co-ordination with university departments of social science:

> Because of the many points of contact between the modern social welfare movement and the public health movement, and to what extent social and economic factors enter into questions of public health, it is clear that an institute of hygiene must take full cognizance of such factors and that students of social science should profit by certain opportunities in the institute, as well as students of hygiene by training in social science and social work.

> The benefits to be expected from the establishment of such an institute as that proposed are not to be measured solely by the number of students trained within its walls. The institute can supply only a relatively small number of those who desire to enter the public health service. The far-reaching influence of the institute should be felt in the advancement of the science and the improvement of the practice of public health in establishing higher standards and better methods of professional education in this field, in stimulating the foundation of similar institutes in other parts of the country, in supplying teachers, and in co-operating with schools of a simpler character designed for briefer technical training which should be established in each state in connection jointly with boards of health and medical schools.

The ideals expressed or implied in the short passages quoted above have not all been realised, but they bore fruit in a development of great importance. When the School of Johns Hopkins was well established, it became a centre for intensive study in special subjects. It frequently happens that a man receives his diploma and goes out into the world to discover, some years later, that he has a special interest in one aspect of his work, or that the conditions of the district in which he is stationed require detailed knowledge of a single subject or group of subjects. He may, for example, desire to undertake an intensive course of study in statistics, in biochemistry, or in clinical subjects such as tuberculosis or venereal disease. It is the privilege of a School of Hygiene to provide instruction in such subjects and to encourage the student to pursue this work to the top of his bent.

In Britain, after the Second World War, there was a very complete review of the position of public health teaching, partly on account of the changing circumstances in the health service due to the National Health Act and partly to the need for evaluation of social medicine as a subject for teaching and practical study by the student. During this period a number of reports were issued, some of them of great interest and practical value. The most complete of these was the report of the Committee on Medical Teaching known as the Goodenough Committee. The Committee began by pointing out that there is no generally accepted definition of social medicine, but they include under that heading the subject of disease prevention. It signifies, they say, a conception of medicine that regards the promotion of health as a primary duty of the doctor, that pays heed to man's social environment and heredity as they affect health, and that recognises the fact that personal problems of health and sickness may have communal aspects. The Committee then go on to say that the training most students receive at the present time is not sufficiently directed towards health and that teaching on the promotion of health and the prevention of disease is often perfunctory and divorced from the rest of the student's curriculum. They point out that the General Medical Council included among the recommendations which it adopted in 1936 this paragraph:

> Throughout the whole period of study, the attention of the student should be directed by his teachers (a) to the importance of the measures by which *Normal Health* may be assessed and

maintained, and (b) to the principles and practice of the Prevention of Disease.

The whole trend of the Committee's view is that the teaching of social and preventive medicine deserves further encouragement so that students and practitioners may have a better knowledge of the influence of social, occupational, genetic and domestic factors on the incidence of human disease and disability. At this point the Goodenough Report refers to the fact that the Royal College of Physicians had published a report on very much the same lines as their own and they agreed that if students are to be fitted to become health advisers in a new national health service, the ideals of social medicine should permeate the whole of medical education. The Committee go even further, and demand a new orientation of medical education, a big expansion in the social work of teaching hospitals, and fundamental changes in outlook and methods of most of the teachers. After dealing with the reorientation of the pre-clinical studies, the Committee specifically recommend that during the clinical period the student's training should include:

(a) appropriate emphasis throughout his clinical studies on the social and preventive aspects;

(b) personal investigations of social and industrial conditions; and

(c) instruction on the communal and administrative sides of disease prevention, on the history of preventive medicine and the evolution of the medical and social services.

The Goodenough Committee then go on to consider this in some detail. They point out, for example, that the fact that a person has fallen ill may be due to causes associated with home conditions, work, or even the way in which he uses his leisure; that his recovery may be hastened or kept back by his mental state, and that his full restoration to health may depend on such matters as the social circumstances to which he returned after discharge from active medical treatment or the opportunities for rehabilitation.

On the second point the Committee urge that students, when acting as medical clerks, should be required to select one or more patients and visit their homes under the guidance of the general practitioner so as to be able to follow them up and make a 'social diagnosis'.

The third comment of the Committee deserves to be reproduced in detail:

The student should learn something of the communal and administrative aspects of preventive medicine and should acquire an elementary knowledge of the duties and responsibilities of a medical officer of health. By this means he can be led to appreciate that prevention is a communal as well as an individual problem, and to realise the ways in which a general practitioner can help the medical officer of health and the public health authority, and in turn can be helped by them in his own practice. His understanding of these matters and of social medicine generally is likely to be aided if he is given a short, elementary account of the development of the medical and social services, of their relation to the social structure and of how progress in the promotion of health has been hindered by such evils as bad housing, ignorance, unemployment, and destitution. The historical approach can be a source of inspiration to the student.

The Committee then discuss who should be responsible for this teaching and they, of course, recognise that it would take time to develop, as well as effort and goodwill. They suggest that each school should make experimental arrangements as soon as possible, and then they set out the suggestion that whatever may be their exact form the arrangements should be designed—

(a) to secure an adequate organisation and integration of the teaching of social medicine in all its aspects;

(b) to achieve the closest possible liaison between the medical school and its hospitals on the one hand, and various outside agencies and persons on the other. These outside agencies and persons include local public health departments, social welfare departments of local authorities, factory doctors, local officers of the Ministry of Health and the Ministry of Labour and National Service, various voluntary organisations, and general practitioners of the district in connection with the visits of students to patients;

(c) to enlist the wholehearted interest and co-operation of the general body of teachers;

(d) to develop and utilise to the full for teaching purposes the social welfare departments of teaching hospitals, and particularly the almoner's department;

(e) to build up an adequate students' health service;

(f) to encourage and facilitate, wherever practicable, the training in matters of health and preventive medicine of school teachers and other non-medical persons without whose intelligent collaboration the promotion of the health of the community cannot be fully achieved.

The Committee then express their belief that their principal objectives could not be achieved unless there was someone on the staff of the medical school whose main interest and responsibility was the furtherance of teaching and research in social medicine and who was free to devote a considerable amount of time to this task.

After dealing with this aspect of the subject, the Committee go on to consider the arrangements for teaching public health. They state the facts but do not draw any conclusions, though they seem to feel that public health is essentially a postgraduate study.

This leads us to the second part of the Committee's report, in which they deal broadly with postgraduate training. Under the heading of public health (p. 219) the Committee limit themselves to a few general observations as follows:

Intending public health officers should add to their general clinical experience by holding appointments as senior house officers in general or special hospitals and by spending some time in general practice. The course of instruction for the postgraduate diploma must be properly planned, and conducted only at institutions that have staff and facilities of university standard. The examination for the diploma should be conducted by the universities providing the training. The final stages of the postgraduate training and experience of the future health officer will presumably consist of service as a member of the staff of a recognised public health department.

Special provision should be made for instruction in industrial medicine and it is a matter for consideration whether this should form an optional part of the public health course or be organised separately.

It will be necessary for the universities generally to raise the standard of the postgraduate training which they provide in preventive medicine. Broadly speaking, the leading postgraduate schools in, say, the United States of America, are better equipped, better staffed and more fully organised both for postgraduate teaching and research, than their British counterparts, with the notable exception of the London School of Hygiene and Tropical Medicine.

The recommendations of the Royal College of Physicians put

forward in the previous year (1943) were very similar to those of the Goodenough Committee. Those that affect us are as follows:

1. That every medical school should establish a department of social and preventive medicine, the size and scope of the department depending upon the facilities and personnel available.

2. That this department should organise a modernised course in social and preventive medicine and replace the present course in public health, which, as in the clinical subjects, should have a curriculum founded securely on the basic sciences, growing and expanding through the three clinical years.

3. As well as theoretical teaching such a curriculum should bring the student into close touch with the active organisations in the community concerned particularly with preventive medicine—namely the health services provided by the local authorities and the almoner's department within the hospitals.

Professor J. A. Ryle put this very well in his book *Changing Disciplines* in which he set out his own conversion to the faith of prevention with characteristic sincerity:

The whole man and his family are still—or rather should be— the practising physician's charge, but they can no longer be considered in detachment from their total environment or from the larger communities of which they are but a part. Communities, large and small, are now due for a more intimate study and care in respect of their health and sickness, but they, too, cannot be considered in detachment from their total environment and from the individuals and families of which they are composed. The state is in the process of planning for larger measures of direction and organisation and a wide extension of services, but state medicine—like clinical medicine—must in the end be based upon scientific principles and humane understanding. A good social medicine must in fact have its foundations in a sound social pathology.[1]

REFERENCES

[1]Ryle, J. A. (1948): *Changing Disciplines,* Oxford University Press.

[2]Ministry of Health, England and Wales (1925): *Memorandum on the Duties of Medical Officers of Health in England and Wales,* p. 1, London, H.M.S.O.

[3]MacQueen, I. A. G. (1960): *Pub. Hlth. (Lond.),* **24,** 244.

[4]Billroth, *The Medical Sciences in the German Universities.*

[5]Huxley, Julian (1944): *On Living in a Revolution,* p. xii, London: Chatto & Windus.

Chapter 6

THE PHYSICALLY HANDICAPPED

One of the striking advances of the early twentieth century, which goes far to justify its title to being called 'The Age of the Child' has led to the position in which the physically handicapped are no longer objects of occasional charity, or freaks that become the subject of idle comment. Society has accepted an obligation to have regard for their welfare. This broad general proposition is, of course, limited in some countries by lack of funds and facilities for care, and there still lingers in times and places an adverse social attitude towards the cripple. Yet a clear case has now been made in all lands for

1. the study of the causes of physical defect;
2. the early and complete ascertainment of the physically handicapped, leading to
3. earlier, and therefore shorter and more effective treatment, and
4. fuller restoration to normal life, and participation in the work of the community; and
5. the insistent search for, and application of preventive measures.

Numbers: One must begin a study of this kind by achieving a right sense of proportion by finding the facts about crippling, that is, the size of the problem. This is an essential preliminary in some of the developing countries. In estimating numbers one has always to exercise caution, partly because certain categories such as the totally blind demand attention, and partly because on the margins of the physical handicap there are many whose symptoms are vague and of short duration. In some countries these have been brought together into a group called 'the delicate', on the ground that they require only brief periods of special care.

In considering the general situation, the first grouping ought to be according to age, on account of the fact that there are two problems of equal dimensions, when a physical handicap has been diagnosed. The first question is to give special skilled attention to diagnosis and treatment, so that all aspects of the physical defect are dealt with. The second matter, of no less importance, is education.

One does not get equality of opportunity when there is only a single track leading from the primary school to the university. The principle has to be accepted that every child should receive the education best suited to his age, ability and aptitude In most countries we have long departed from the idea that education is required only for the professions and for leadership in politics. In modern times the new educational needs are not least for the benefit of ordinary people, so that they may learn to understand the society in which we live. 'A community that is committed to adult suffrage is committed also either to rich, diverse, and efficient education or to chaos.'[1] Equality thus means diversity of opportunity; and considerations of this kind have vital consequences for physically handicapped children. It means that they must no longer be cast aside as misfits, but that each child should be considered as a potential entrant to the ordinary school. We do NOT want diluted education—a weak, aqueous solution of the teaching given to the bright child—but the right adjustment to the actual needs of the handicapped, the method, subject, emphasis, and class organisation. A system tolerating large classes and poor conditions of learning produces children who, in addition to their physical handicap, are educationally disabled. The work of assessment and the educational decision, or placement, ought not to rest on the teaching side alone; the school health officer has an important part to play, because he has not only the task of judging capacity but has a duty through such expert medical advice and care as can be obtained to apply treatment and to modify the child's way of life in such a manner as to enable the child to achieve as high a degree of normality as the physical handicap allows.

If we take as a rough guide a figure of 800 per 100,000 registered pupils as representing the physically handicapped—with the exception of those suffering solely from a defect of sight or hearing—then this group covers the children who by reason of disease or crippling defect cannot be satisfactorily educated under the normal regime of ordinary schools. The distribution obviously varies from one country to another and at different periods of time, but in England around 1950 it had the following percentage of all the handicapped as defined above:

Poliomyelitis	18	Cerebral palsy	9
Osteomyelitis	4	Congenital disability	24
Tuberculosis of bone and		Injuries	10
joint	3	Arthritis, flat-foot, scoli-	
Rickets	2	osis, kyphosis, etc.	30

Today these conditions make up in the main the 'orthopedic' defects which, 'whether arising from deformity, disease, or accident, give rise to a functional disability of the organs of locomotion.' The essentials of orthopedic care are:

1. General preventive measures, such as specific teaching in schools and through television, the press, and other methods of publicity. For example, an untrained child on a faulty bicycle is an accident on its way to happen.

2. Early and accurate ascertainment. An attempt to deal with a problem of this sort without getting the facts and knowing even the extent of the question to be answered is like setting out on a voyage without a compass.

3. Prompt and effective *early* care at a clinic, with the primary object of avoiding the need for hospitalisation, or at least to secure a substantial reduction of hospital treatment.

4. Where necessary in view of the condition of the child, specialised hospital treatment for the acute phase; and long-term physical and educational care in a residential hospital school.

5. Education in the hospital, integrated with treatment and not casually introduced.

6. A chain of accessible clinics for intermediate care and follow-up by the expert staff of the hospital.

7. So far as necessary on educational grounds, or as a result of long stay in hospital, vocational training for children and adolescents.

ASCERTAINMENT

An efficient scheme depends first and last on early and accurate ascertainment. If there is a time delay, one or both of two consequences are liable to happen: (a) minor disabilities are missed altogether, and in the course of time are likely to become major handicaps; (b) more serious defects, neglected early, tend to become permanent. Moreover, treatment becomes progressively more difficult and more prolonged—and less sure in its results. From the more general administrative point of view lack of ascertainment gives a false picture of the incidence of physical defects; it thus tends to produce in the authorities a sense of complacency in the belief that they are dealing with all the existing cases, when in fact they are probably becoming aware mainly of the less curable patients.

It is a very difficult matter to ascertain the number of crippled children who are not in fact attending school, as they are often not entered in the registers of the school authorities. Some, unhappily, are in hospital without receiving any education at all; others are being deliberately withheld by their parents, either as a result of ill-conceived affection, trying in vain to shield them from life's difficulties; or for less reputable reasons such as prestige, or ignorance, in the belief that no education is possible. What then is to be done for the disabled children of parents who, for good or indifferent motives, fail to take advantage of facilities for medical and educational care? Parental rights are respected in democratic countries by faith, law and tradition. The incursion of the State into the home would be met with antagonism, even for such beneficent purposes as the physical and mental welfare of the children. Nevertheless, it is not conceivable that contemporary society should allow children to suffer neglect, even when the obstruction to care is well motivated and when it is protected by the recognised sanctity of the home. Children, as Alva Myrdal put it, are the unenfranchised citizens of tomorrow,[2] and their elders have social as well as parental duties towards them. It would be against public opinion, and perhaps against the public interest, to compel parents to send their children to hospitals or schools for the physically disabled; but it would surely be reasonable to require that the appropriate health and education authorities be *informed* of the presence of a disabled child. Notification by a medical practitioner should be required as soon as he becomes aware, for it is only mistaken kindness to wait. There should also be a duty laid upon hospitals to notify the health authorities. What happens after that is a matter for personal guidance and understanding.

PREVENTIVE CARE

There are two aspects of preventive work: the first consists of a broad programme of health education, which is best undertaken by co-operative enterprise between voluntary bodies and the health authorities. In addition, more specific health education and demonstration is widely undertaken, by contacts with maternal and child health centres, nursery schools, and all grades of school; and also more directly with the public through meetings and conferences, press information, and radio and television. Television is particularly valuable as a medium for the presentation of such subjects as the prevention of accidents, and the press for drawing constant attention to accidents which have occurred, and laying stress on the preventive aspects and on what might be done to avoid recurrences.

The second aspect of the programme is the provision of skilled care at the earliest possible moment, so that the original damage may not be intensified by delay or unskilled handling. This applies especially to the organisation *in advance* of emergency arrangements with hospitals and clinics to deal with accidents. In this connection one cannot praise too highly the hospital disaster services which have now been developed over wide areas, and the co-operation between hospitals and other authorities which this implies. Other matters of moment, discussed elsewhere, include special training in first aid and resuscitation as a protection against drowning and similar accidents, and the establishment of first aid posts in particularly dangerous areas. Apart from accident protection, one must not forget the other preventive services in which special skill and early attention is essential. It has been pointed out that large numbers of physical handicaps arise in early infancy or during the ante-natal period. This has been tragically illustrated several times in recent years, but particularly in the case of ante-natal deformities associated with the drug thalidomide. There is no need to enlarge on this as it received such widespread publicity in 1962; but the lesson to be drawn is that the authorities must be constantly on the lookout for disasters of this kind. Some of them indeed may be occurring at frequent intervals but as yet unrecognised owing largely to our lack of knowledge of the conditions at this critical stage of pregnancy which affect the growing foetus. There is an urgent need for two major moves throughout the world. The first is to secure critical reassessment of drugs liable to be taken by pregnant women, and the second is to make sure that no conditions of this kind are escaping notice owing to lack of knowledge or want of attention on the part of science and medicine.

Many of the physical defects which so arise are most readily and effectively treated in infancy, when the tissues are pliable and so respond well to non-operative treatment such as correction by moulding and subsequent use of plaster. The aim is to avoid the need for hospital care by saving a limb from deformity at the earliest moment.

HOSPITAL TREATMENT

In the fully developed orthopedic hospital scheme there are two principal phases: the acute, and the long-term (or post-acute). The acute cases consist mainly of fractures and urgent illness, and many of these are dealt with directly in the special surgical units of the great hospitals, with a possible transfer to the long-term hospital for subsequent care and restoration. For long term patients the most desirable accommodation for children is the hospital school in country surroundings. This does not necessarily indicate that the unit should be remote from populous areas; but it does emphatically imply that it should be surrounded by fresh air, trees and grass, and free from noise, bustle and smoke of city life. The essential features are community life, education according to capacity, occupation, and fun. There should be ample provision for outdoor recreation for both patients and staff; but perhaps the most important need of all is continuity. In one country orthopedic hospital with which I was associated considerable attention was given to education of children, and in co-operation with the local authority a regular teaching staff was organised for the service. Daily lessons were given at the bedside, and in suitable cases there was a certain amount of 'homework' which generally consisted of reading literature. In the course of time it was

F

observed that certain difficulties had arisen, chiefly due to a
sub-conscious clash between teaching and nursing staff.
Naturally enough, the nursing and the younger surgical staff
felt that treatment should always take the first place and that
teaching was a secondary consideration, useful no doubt for
filling in the time. The teachers, on the other hand, began to
feel that they were being pushed around to suit the convenience
of all other personnel, and were more or less interlopers. The
action finally taken was drastic enough, but it solved the
difficulties. The hospital authority set up a series of separate
school-rooms, and it was arranged that all children who could
possibly benefit should be wheeled in beds or chairs to the
school-room. This became part of the duty of the hospital
staff, with the help of the more active adult and child patients.
And it was agreed that, wherever possible, patients who were
due to be seen by the surgical staff should be notified to the
teachers, and sent for treatment in good time. The usual ward
round was held at a definite time which would not interfere
with the school periods. This apparently complicated arrangement had many advantages in practice. It was popular with
nurses because it enabled them to have more time to spend in
the morning and afternoon on the patients who really needed
skilled   attention—without   constant   interruption   from
clamorous youngsters who had become accustomed to order
the staff around. The plan was also highly popular with the
wardmaids, because it enabled them to clean the floors and
attend to their other duties, again with much more freedom and
effectiveness in the relatively empty wards. At first the younger
surgical staff felt at a loss, due to the fact that they had become
used to turning up at all hours. Now they found that punctuality
of attendance was the only sound way of getting good service
from the nursing staff, and of making comprehensive rounds in
preparation for the senior surgeons. The latter could, of course,
call for a particular patient at any time, as of right; so no
trouble arose in their august ranks.

Rather unexpectedly, the children also preferred the new
system. The admission to a definite 'school' gave them a sense
of prestige, of being something more than sick children. They
became very proud of their school, as it gave them that delight-
ful feeling of independence from the unending routine of the

hospital ward. Further, the children made better progress under school discipline and, like most normal children, they enjoyed the school routines and the companionships created. In a similar way, the existence of a separate school made the play of these children much more meaningful, and at the same time it was possible for both teaching and medical staff to join together in watching progress in physical activities, and in noting for consultation any points that seemed to require surgical intervention, limitation, or guidance.

FOLLOW UP AND AFTER CARE

When a patient leaves the hospital, his treatment has not been completed. It may have only just commenced. The ideal is not merely the correction of deformities or the provision of apparatus; it is the restoration of function. This is the reason why special stress must always be laid on the value of having expert staff on the spot from the very beginning of the disability at the clinic to make the right start and to secure continuity of care. It is therefore of great importance that parents should bring the child at regular intervals to one of the hospital clinics until final discharge. It is no less important that educational follow up should also be undertaken, so as to keep a steady watch on the child's aptitudes and progress. The greatest harm is often done by underestimating the child's capacities, and confusing the handicap of the body with the condition and possibilities of the mind. This is particularly applicable to children suffering from cerebral palsy, because their physical disability is often so obvious as to conceal the real educational capacity of the child.

Physically handicapped children who are intellectually suitable for higher school education and college sometimes present difficulties to the authorities when, owing to the need for active treatment, they miss the occasion of the selection test; or perhaps when they are not ready at the usual age, on account of prolonged hospital care. On the other hand, the difficulty may arise because of their failure to be accepted for the higher schools, even after selection on intelligence grounds. The reason given would usually be a doubt as to whether they could stay the course on account of physical defect, or possibly that the school or college buildings were unsuitable for the safe handling of cripples (e.g., due to steep and narrow stairways).

In a survey made of English Grammar School buildings it was found that the actual building construction varied from old buildings of several storeys and, of course, without lifts, to single storey bungalows. Even with this, most of the schools had awkward steps here and there. No schools of this kind had in fact any special facilities for dealing with the physically handicapped, such as ramps or lifts. In practice it was remarkable to notice how many of the supposed hazards were ignored or overcome by the crippled. Generally speaking, the more serious defects in construction were concerned with toilet accommodation, but in fact this difficulty was readily surmounted through the eager help of other pupils, and the appointment, week by week, of special 'monitors' from the various classes. In some schools, class rooms on the ground floor were redesignated for the teaching of the handicapped children, but of course not as separate groups. In some areas children were rejected if they were not able to go unaided to the toilet; or if they were unable to sit up and had to spend the day in a semi-supine position; and lastly, if they required a wheeled chair and there were many steps to be negotiated. It was found that the most important responsibility was to be sure that the handicapped child was not left alone too long, for example, when the others were out at play. The distress experienced by an immobile pupil, when left alone, may be severe. On the whole, however, the problems which had seemed fearsome worked out quite well in practice. Probably the greatest difficulty, fortunately rare, was incontinence. Discipline was the same for all, and independence has to be taught without creating overstrain, as when the crippled child has to be taught to *watch* games. He should not be expected to do extra study while the others are playing.

The great majority of handicapped children who were taught in the higher schools under these conditions were happy. It gave them much pleasure and satisfaction. They made every effort to keep up with the pace, and the very last thing they wanted was to be considered as 'handicapped'. A few boys and girls were demanding or self-pitying, and tended to exploit their misfortune. Most of them improved after a frank talk with an understanding master. If, as occasionally happened, a single child required a helper all the time, it was vital that this help be given on a rota system, so as to avoid any one pupil being overwhelmed by the handicapped child—and no complaint against either of them. But in the end it is the courage of the cripple that calls out the best in his fellow-pupils.

THE BLIND

From the educational point of view the blind are defined as pupils who have no sight or whose sight is, or is likely to become, so defective that they require education by methods not involving the use of sight. The number in England and Wales is about 20 per 100,000 registered pupils. The incidence has decreased since the end of the first world war, due to (a) the decline of ophthalmia neonatorum from 28% to 5% of blind children, and (b) the reduction of interstitial keratitis from 8% to 2%. On the other hand we have to keep a sharp eye on the world picture and the great scourges that lead to blindness.

Practically every blind child must be educated in a special school, so that it is not necessary to enter into any teaching details. There are, however, one or two special features of the group which refer to public health care, notably some psychological effects that are not widely understood. The Scottish Department (Cmd. 7885: HMSO) put the matter well: 'Nightfall brings to the sighted an ever-recurring reminder of the problems of the blind. Colours are drained from the world by every twilight; shapes assume an unfamiliar vagueness; movements become mere hints of change in the surroundings. These experiences are interpreted by normal people, no matter how devoid of vision they may be, in the light of *visual* memories. They convey only a feeble impression of the world of the blind, but they are sufficient to prompt a concern for those whose days are spent in perpetual darkness.' It is noteworthy that the author, Graham Greene, who builds a fortress of unexampled callousness around his character of 'the Boy', has to admit one, and only one, chink in the wall: it is when 'the boy' discovers that he has been pushing roughly aside a group of blind musicians—not realising that they were blind. There is a note of faint regret for his action.

The main psychological features that are apt to arise in blind children are:

1. The risk of verbalism; that is, of using words and phrases disembodied of reality. Our object in the darkening days is to enlarge their experience even at the expense of their vocabulary.

2. Social adjustments. Blindness may become an occasion for selfishness or for self-mastery. The blind child, especially if kept too long at home, may exploit his disability to create a tyranny—while in school he is more likely to seek comradeship and understanding.

3. Self-pity, leading to day-dreaming and so into the vicious circle of total isolation, from which removal is exceedingly difficult.

4. 'Blindisms' constitute a psycho-physical habit of spasms and grotesque gestures which a seeing child would readily correct. It is by no means easy to make similar corrections in the blind child.

5. The value of concentration on the things of the mind, such as literature or music, as a partial compensation for the lost visual arts. It is not necessarily good for the blind 'to learn tricks' that would be normal actions in a seeing person.

6. Psychological compensation. In order to explain the full and useful lives that many of the blind live, a theory has been put forward that they can develop certain compensations—a special sensitivity of hearing or touch, a kind of sixth sense which enables them to locate obstacles in their path. The idea is certainly a tribute to the remarkable cleverness of many blind persons, but the facts do not support it. Careful research has shown no special sensitivity of memory consciousness; but many of the blind do undoubtedly accumulate a group of sensory clues which help them to avoid objects—just as a seeing person learns how to get out of his garage! There is reason to believe, for example, that the blind can learn to become very sensitive to certain temperature and pressure changes when they are very close to surfaces such as walls or stationary vehicles (Cmd. 7885, p. 17). This enables them to move along streets and lobbies with some confidence and to recognise the places at which the street wall comes to an end, presumably at a crossing. One of the most recent comments about blindness was a kindly caution from a blind person not to seize the blind

by the arm, but rather to allow the blind to take the guiding person's arm. This, it was stated, gave a much greater sense of confidence, because it had not the unpleasant 'imprisoning' effect.

THE PARTIALLY SIGHTED

In the record previously referred to the total category of the partially sighted amounted to about 100 per 100,000 registered pupils. There are considerable variations in assessment, however, between one country and another, depending partly on medical and educational diagnosis and partly on the special accommodation available. In any case many of the partially sighted can and should be educated in an ordinary classroom beside sighted children. Good lighting, both natural and artificial, is essential, and a favourable position in class. The pupil must be able to see easily both the teacher and the blackboard. One should not lay too much emphasis on writing or reading from books, or even the blackboard, unless it is well lighted. Partially sighted children vary a great deal in their needs: some require a very dark, thick pencil and the use of a bold script, while others, with an equal handicap, can manage ordinary writing and may reach grammar school level. The test for education in the ordinary school is simple enough, viz: progress in the primary school, more than actual or potential vision. Much depends on what we may call 'visual skill'; that is, the intelligent use of vision.

In England before 1944 a partially sighted child was classified as blind, but under the Act of that year the definition has been greatly improved and now reads: 'pupils who, by reason of defective vision, cannot follow the ordinary curriculum without detriment to their sight or to their educational development, but can be educated by special methods involving the use of sight.' And so partially sighted children are no longer in the country of the blind and can, with a few exceptions, enjoy many of the normal activities and interests of children of their own age.

Ascertainment: Much depends on the primary cause. If it is an error of refraction, the primary cause is mainly myopia and myopic astigmatism. The second group consists of inflammation resulting from injury or infection, and giving rise to scarring, especially of the cornea. There may, on the other hand, be a congenital defect, or progressive degeneration of the optic nerve or the retina. The percentage of myopes in special schools has varied from 30 to 75, and a good deal of controversy has arisen about their place in special schools. In these, as in special classes, the emphasis is on sight saving, and the risks of detachment of the retina have been given prominence. This is now rare, and many ophthalmologists doubt the value of undue restrictions. Even if, by excessive care, one could save a few dioptres or a few months of sight, is it worth while?

This raises the principle of the major defect, that is, of sight saving versus the richer content of education. Surely it is of the utmost importance that an intelligent child should receive adequate preparation for the darkness to come.

There is no hard and fast test for admission to a special school, but it has been suggested as follows:

1. Fundus changes as indicating serious myopia.

2. In the absence of the above, on repeated examination, a steady increase of more than one dioptre a year; or, after a period of slow increase, a sudden rise to more than one dioptre a year.

3. The younger the child, the more serious the condition.

4. In non-myopics, a visual acuity after correction of 6/24 or worse, with a near vision of J8 or J10 (i.e., 6/24-6/60 in the better eye).

5. One should take general progress into account, and have teamwork to ascertain intelligence, health, psychological attitude, etc.

6. A child should not be educated as a blind pupil simply because at some time in the future he will need to make use of Braille.

THE DEAF

The blind attract the sympathy of ordinary people more readily than the deaf, for the reason that it requires more imaginative understanding to appreciate the solitary mental life of the deaf in an unfamiliar world. The world of people, as of things, is known in a limited way only by the deaf child. 'When he is left alone at night there are no comforting echoes of familiar voices to share his loneliness; when his mother passes beyond his range of vision, she disappears with an abruptness that does not occur in the life of a hearing child. The deaf child has a double handicap in his relation to the world of things: his loss of hearing limits his experience of material things, and his impaired powers of communication reduce his chances of learning from the world of men.'[3]

The estimates of the number of deaf children in England is about 70 per 100,000 registered pupils. By this is meant pupils who have no hearing or whose hearing is so defective that they require education by methods used for deaf pupils without naturally acquired speech or language. This does not necessarily include those who have lost hearing after acquiring speech or language, made habitual by use.

The term 'deaf and dumb' tends to hide the most serious handicap of children born deaf. Even the most talkative of us would choose to retain hearing rather than speech. The untaught deaf child is not only deaf and dumb, but also WORDLESS, which is far worse. If we habitually think without words, our vocabulary is very limited, and even more so the range of thought. When we lack words, then even the simplest books are closed to us. For this reason, the chief aim lies in teaching the child to gain knowledge of words, so that he can use them in thinking, in comprehending through lip-reading the speech of other people, and, through vibrations, learning the art of speech, and finally of reading and writing. In the case of the severely handicapped by partial deafness we must use every means, including the residual hearing capacity, to increase and make accurate the child's knowledge of his native language. Thus it is clear that the prime need of a deaf child who has lost hearing is to be helped to retain the use of speech learned while he could hear, and enabled to make contact, through normal language, with normal people. This means in practice adding daily to the store of words and making use of even the slightest residue of hearing which, from nine months onwards, can be developed by means of hearing aids. Speech is the strongest link in human fellowship and in the social relations of man.

The successful training of a wordless child depends on:

1. his general intelligence;
2. his behaviour—a very real difficulty in deaf children;

3. his residual capacity, if any;
4. eyesight (for lip-reading etc.);
5. physique.

'Deaf-mutism' is an unpopular but descriptive term. It inevitably follows deafness in less than ten years unless the child has been suitably educated. The older child, when he is stricken with deafness, follows the same course, and even more quickly. In fact, even at the upper school limit most children entirely lose their speech within six months, unless they are trained. Heredity seems to account for some 60% of deaf children, and non-heredity, prenatal conditions around 5%, in the congenital group. Of the acquired group post-meningeal deafness gives another 20% and other forms 15%. Children born deaf seldom have an absolute loss, but their hearing is usually patchy and small. They are seldom able to profit by hearing aids. Postmeningeal deafness often follows quite mild attacks of the disease and is the commonest change except personality. The child is often unstable and has personality problems. The deafness does not necessarily follow the acute illness immediately, but progresses insidiously after discharge from hospital, sometimes resulting in total deafness. This often leads to intolerable delays in securing the urgently necessary education, bringing anguish to the misunderstood child, because he is thought to be merely stupid. It is therefore essential that there should be the closest co-operation between the hospital, the school teacher and the school health service, and full-tone audiograms should be taken every two months for two years in the case of a child who gives a history of 'meningitis' or the mother gives an account of a similar complaint. Under good hospital care less than half are deaf on discharge; but these children become rapidly mute or, if only partially deaf, show diminished educational performance, unless special education is begun at once. Acquired deafness of this nature should be regarded as a medical emergency—like diabetes for example. The child should on no account be permitted a time of waiting, e.g., until a new term begins. If immediate school attendance is not possible, then home teaching should begin at once. The ordinary process of ascertainment should be cut short by the school health officer.

The education of the deaf child begins as soon as the diagnosis is made, by home teaching, even at less than one year. The child should be sent to school as early as possible, preferably at three to four years. The ideal system is a boarding school, with the week-ends at home, except towards school leaving age, when day school may be substituted. To continue with boarding all the time makes the child rather vulnerable to the harsh outside world, and further, it interferes with the proper and necessary education of the child's *family*.

As far as educational methods are concerned, the experts and enthusiasts have set themselves the ideal of an end-product of their teaching who can communicate by lip-reading and speech with hearing persons in the ordinary social intercourse of life. They therefore lay great stress on lip-reading and speech training. They deprecate sign language as being undignified, useless as a method of communication with the general public, leading to short cuts and making real training more difficult. Some children learn lip-reading more quickly than others, and speech is easier for those who have heard. For those born deaf the ability to lip-read is not closely related to intelligence or educability. Even more important is that (except for the few) it takes so long to lip-read and speak with hearing persons in the ordinary social intercourse of life that elementary education is severly retarded. If the child is taught by sign language as a supplement to visual means, it at least makes it possible for deaf children to communicate with one another, and this is good fun! It would be fantastic to forbid it.

A vitally important feature of the education of the deaf child is to make sure that his family is trained to make the best of the situation. It is distressing to see a deaf child home for the week-end, with no means of communicating with his family except goo-goo language. No one ever troubles to teach the parents to lip-read, or use sign language. As often as not even the mother has no real channel of communication and is apt to accept baby language as a matter of sentimentality. The brothers and sisters become bored with what they would feel to be an unco-operative playmate. When the deaf child goes to school, both parents should be trained in communication and understanding. Deaf children are apt to suffer from tantrums. This often arises from sheer exasperation at not being under-stood, and so a number of the major behaviour problems can be eliminated by simple training of the other members of the family group. There is also need for the examination of the eyes of the deaf child as a routine, because of the risk that retinitis pigmentosa or congenital cataract may be missed.

One should always think of the possibility of deafness in investigating behaviour problems in a child. Deaf infants babble like normal babies up to about seven months. Then, as they get no satisfaction from bigger and better babbles, they tend to lapse into silence. This may be succeeded by toneless, raucous sounds and grunts to attract adult attention. These weird noises are often the first indication that medical advice is necessary.

THE PARTIALLY DEAF

The partially deaf are estimated at about 100 per 100,000, but few require special school education. The group is defined as pupils who have some naturally acquired speech and language, but whose hearing is so defective that they require for their education special arrangements or facilities, though not necessarily all the educational methods needful for deaf children. Articulation may be faulty; vocabulary limited, speech childish; but the child can be taught to hear enough with an aid to be taught orally. Early ascertainment is paramount; and the earlier the hearing aid is brought into use the more likely is it to be accepted by the child—even before twelve months. Where children become deaf after speech has been acquired, the importance of immediate instruction in lip-reading cannot be overestimated. Then the children, especially if they are intelligent, can generally make good progress in ordinary schools—perhaps after a short period of adjustment. The special school or classroom should be quiet, away from street noises. Whether the pupil goes to a special school or not depends not on hearing loss, but on whether the child has had the opportunity or the capacity to acquire speech. If, after six months in an ordinary school, the child fails to maintain clear speech and comprehension of what is said, then a special school is advisable.

Of children who become deaf 62% are so before two years, 22% between two and five years, and 5% between five and nine years. A child who *has* heard, even down to nine months of age, has an advantage over the child born deaf. This lies in the cumulative experience of voices, speech, and the incidental sounds associated with them. When illness at less than nine months deprives a child of hearing, memories and associations fade quickly, but some progress can be held by skilled training, and so prevent a total lapse. If no training at all is given, a considerable number of those who become deaf at two to three years of age become dumb as well at four to five years old. Children of this group need both training and encouragement because the grave 'shock of silence' in children under five is not so serious at later years, as the children can understand the position better. As has been noted, special school teachers in general frown on the use of the deaf alphabet; but used within reason it has a definite play value, as it can readily be learned by both children and adults. It is also a language of fun among deaf children who want to communicate, e.g., in a poor light. In England there was a recent appeal from more than two thousand deaf people to restore the use of the alphabet—and one must not be too doctrinaire on the subject.

REFERENCES

[1]LOWNDES, A. M.: *The Silent Social Revolution.*
[2]MYRDAL, ALVA (1941): *Nation and Family*, p. 237, New York and London, Harper Bros.
[3]Scottish Department of Health. Cmd. 7885.

Chapter 7

MENTAL HEALTH
IN PUBLIC HEALTH PRACTICE

In its historical background the mental health service has a good deal in common with other developments in preventive medicine. It would have entered the field earlier, but for the unfortunate defect in the public (and frequently the professional) outlook on mental disorder. In addition, many countries which were advanced in other respects still clung to the age-long association of mental disorder and defect with the stigma of poverty. It was not until the nineteenth century that the legal provision of special accommodation for the 'insane' was secured. Private asylums had been in existence for many years previously, but the fate of their inmates was commonly worse than in the public institutions. The stigma attaching to mental disease was so gross that the keeper of a private home could extract large fees for hiding away the skeleton in the family cupboard.

In medieval times the apparatus for the care of the mentally ill was simple. A Royal Commission investigating the conditions of the famous Bethlem Hospital in London in 1403 recorded the inventory of fittings as including: '6 chains of iron with 6 locks; 4 pairs of mannicles of iron, and 2 pairs of stocks.' In these early days, however, only the violent patients were chained and the harmless were allowed to wander around the city, begging for alms. During the seventeenth and early eighteenth centuries this hospital became a show-place, and charges for admission to see the inmates were said to realise as much as four hundred pounds a year. Bethlem was closed to sightseers in 1770, and from then onwards the patients were no longer regarded as wild animals on show and began to enjoy the blessings and amenities of medical treatment. The routine summarised by the visiting physician at the beginning of the nineteenth century was as follows:

Patients are ordered to be bled about the latter end of May, according to the weather, and after that had been completed, they take vomits once a week for a certain number of weeks. After that we purge our patients. This has been the practice invariably for years, long before my time; it was handed down to me by my father, and I do not know of any better practice.

By this time the physician might well have looked around, even at his own country, and certainly in France. In England the first step in progress was taken by William Tuke, a Quaker citizen of York, who founded the institution called 'The Retreat', in which humane treatment was substituted for coercion and physical restraint. In the early nineteenth century pioneers in mental hospitals in European and North American countries followed similar methods. In many cases, however, the law was slow to follow the lead given by the pioneer, and the nineteenth century records a hard struggle between the old, crowded, prison-like institutions and the advanced hospitals. Another hindrance to development arises from the persistent association *in the public mind* of mental disorder with compulsory detention, and the clumsy process of certification as a necessary preliminary to treatment. Although these associations are no longer valid in the advancing countries, the idea often persists in the public mind that the mental hospital is a place for compulsory and indefinite incarceration. This belief cannot be broken down by changes in the law alone, because some degree of compulsory power must be retained for a small minority of cases, for the protection of the public. It can be counteracted in two ways: by the education of the people to realise that the mental hospital is an institution specially designed for the care of persons suffering from illness; and by giving every encouragement for the ready acceptance of treatment on a voluntary basis.

The value of the law as a preventive has been considered elsewhere, and it is just as necessary in the sphere of mental illness as in any other department of public health. Nevertheless, while elaborate legal precautions against wrongful detention serve to ease the minds of the public, these very safeguards may deter sensitive patients and their families from seeking the benefits of early treatment. The Report of the Commission on Lunacy and Mental Disorder (England, 1926) urged that the intervention of the law should be as unobtrusive as possible:

To over-emphasise the legal aspect of the treatment of mental disease would in our view only tend to perpetuate the idea of imprisonment with which insanity has been too long associated, and to increase its differentiation from other illnesses.

This Report is a good illustration of the revolution in the attitude towards mental treatment since the end of the nineteenth century. As the Report itself says:

With the advance of medical science and the growth of more enlightened views, insanity is coming to be regarded from an entirely different stand-point. It is being perceived that insanity is, after all, only a disease like other diseases, though with definite symptoms of its own, and that a mind diseased can be ministered to no less effectively than a body diseased. But the old conception of insanity dies hard and its traits are still persistent. The modern conception calls for the eradication of old social prejudices and the complete revision of the attitude of society in the matter of its duty towards the mentally afflicted.

The main principles which determined the proposals that the Commission brought forward were summarised in the following bold phrases:

The treatment of mental disorder should approximate as nearly to the treatment of physical ailments as is consistent with the special safeguards which are indispensable when the liberty of the subject is infringed. Certification should be the last resort and not a necessary preliminary to treatment. The procedure for certification should be simplified and made uniform for private and publicly supported cases alike, and dissociated from the Poor Laws.

The Statute which followed the Report of the Commission of 1926 introduced advances in law and practice of far-reaching importance. On the clinical side the most effective provisions were the creation of two new categories: voluntary patients and temporary patients. The former included all patients who were able to express an opinion, and the more restricted provisions of the latter referred to those who were unable to express volition. The procedure for dealing with voluntary patients was simple, and in recent years it has been used in a considerable majority of cases; but the temporary arrangements were hedged round with all sorts of restrictive conditions, because they were based, not on the prospects of recovery, but rather on the legalistic test of volition. Provision for voluntary mental patients without certificate, which had been legal in Scotland since 1866, was ultimately applied alike to the poor and to the well-to-do in England under the Mental Treatment Act of 1930. The success of these measures has led to a more general understanding of the hospital care of the mental patient, and in recent years a great advance has been made, under the Act of 1959, in the application of 'open door' methods of care.

The 1959 Act cleared away a great mass of confusing legislation in both the Lunacy and the Mental Deficiency Acts. The passing of the Act is a recognition of important developments in the general pattern of services, but especially it emphasises services for patients living outside hospitals. Probably the most important change has been that the Statutes now accept the situation that most of the restrictions and restraints used in mental hospitals in the past are now outdated, and that modern psychology applied to the needs of patients creates remarkable improvements in attitude, and the older hostilities and fears largely disappear.

In addition to legislation, however, one must mention that modern physical treatment and new forms of drugs have made great improvements in early care, and have enabled the restoration of chronic patients to be more rapid and successful. The Report of the Chief Medical Officer of the Ministry of Health for the year 1959 states that the resident population of the mental hospitals of England and Wales decreased by 15,000 between 1955 and 1959. This is accounted for by three factors: increased out-patient treatment, reducing the need for admission; earlier and more effective treatment in hospital, lessening the need for prolonged care; and active rehabilitation of long-stay patients, making an increasing number of them either self-supporting or fit for care in the community. (P. 131).

It is of great interest to observe that these simple changes, which have revolutionised the care of mental disorder, are in the main readily applicable to hospital services in the less developed countries. What is more, they could be applied with good effect in hospitals much less elaborate than those that used to be considered essential for mental care. The real concentration in those countries should be not upon hospitals as such, but rather on the services which can be rendered, such as increasing home care, out-patient attendance, the day hospital, and admission to geriatric and other units, according to the assessment of the individual patient.

VOLUNTARY ASSOCIATIONS

In England the first of the voluntary societies specifically related to mental health was the Mental After-Care Association, which was founded in 1879. Its first President was the Earl of Shaftesbury, who had already done so much in this as in other social activities. In those earlier days it was essentially a rehabilitation society designed to bridge the gap between the return of the patient from a mental hospital and the difficulties in adjusting to everyday working life. More recently the Association has been interested in the promotion of convalescent homes and activities of that kind. It will be interesting to follow its development in consequence of recent legislation, especially the change in attitude towards mental illness and the open-door treatment in hospitals. It is almost certain that there will be an increasing need for homes of this kind as an intermediate stage. At any rate the Association has done admirable pioneer work and although its functions were largely confined to the metropolitan area its influence on opinion was far greater.

The Central Association for Mental Welfare was founded in 1913. Its primary objective was to act as a maternity nurse for the Mental Deficiency Act of that year, and to follow it into full operation. The Association gradually developed an excellent scheme for the care of mental defectives (as its original name suggested), through the provision of Occupation Centres and home visiting in close co-operation with local authorities. This was achieved by means of the establishment of Local Voluntary Associations to help in the implementation of the new Act, to initiate statutory and voluntary enterprise under it, and to educate public opinion.

Training was provided for social workers wishing to become Secretaries of Voluntary Associations, and short training courses were held annually for mental deficiency officers on local authority staffs. Courses for School Medical Officers, held in co-operation with the University of London, were inaugurated in 1920 and became thereafter a regular feature of the Association's work.

The first world war created new problems in mental health, partly on account of the stress imposed on people by war conditions. For this reason the National Council for Mental Hygiene was formed, not only to handle local questions but also to deal with the broader problems of international relationships, and in this way to lay the foundation for a world mental health organisation. One of its first tasks was to make a critical study of the psychoneuroses and to provide clinics and services for early mental disorders. It promoted the teaching of psychiatry in medical schools and did much to provide clinical care in general rather than mental hospitals for this class of case. In this way, during the period 1930-40 the Council went far in helping to mould public opinion.

The Child Guidance Council was imported from the United States in 1927, through the very present help of the Commonwealth Fund. Its aim was to provide skilled treatment for children suffering from behaviour disorders. The personal work in England of skilled demonstrations under Miss M. C. Scoville and the fine arrangements made by the Commonwealth Fund for training the early workers from England in the United States ensured a sound beginning. Through this pioneer effort there was a gradual acceptance by the public of the child guidance programme, and in the course of time the Ministry of Education took up the matter as a necessary provision in its schools.

As time went on, each of these organisations extended its functions, and there arose a good deal of overlapping. In 1936 a serious attempt was made to combine. This was promoted by means of a General Reconstruction Committee under the chairmanship of the Earl of Feversham. This Committee had the full support of the Board of Control. The following is an extract from the Annual Report of the Board of Control for the year 1935:

> The fact that the Board's statutory duties are so largely concerned with the institutional care of cases of mental disorder or defect tends to create an impression that their interests and their duties are confined to institutional problems. This is far from being the case. On the contrary, the Board take the view that institutional care is only a part, although admittedly the most costly part, of a health service which includes all aspects of mental

hygiene. The special problems of child guidance, of the treatment of border-line cases, of after-care and preventive care, and the manifold problems, medical, social and educational, associated with mental deficiency are all closely related, and to attempt to deal with them in isolation is neither scientific nor conducive to the most economical use of the available resources. The Board cordially agree with Professor Henderson of Edinburgh when he says (in his report for 1935), 'We must learn to talk of mental health and its maintenance rather than of mental disease and its cure.' Until this is generally recognised no real progress can be made on preventive lines, and sectional interests will continue to compete against one another for public support.

With these considerations in mind the Board have noted with pleasure the growing movement in favour of combining, whether by complete amalgamation or by federation with a central body, all the various voluntary agencies interested in different aspects of mental health. The want of unified direction and a comprehensive central body able to view the problem as a whole has made the mental hygiene movement relatively ineffective in this country. Without some measure of union, or at least of co-ordination, no effective appeal can be made to the public for financial support and, an even graver source of weakness, no real advance can be made in educating public opinion so that the needs and possibilities of the work may be more fully realised. The development of any health service depends upon close co-operation between voluntary effort and governmental or municipal activities. Legislation in advance of public opinion is almost always inoperative, nor can local authorities be criticised for failing to do more than their constituents want them to do. There are limits to the extent to which central departments can influence or, indeed, ought to attempt to influence public opinion. It is therefore all the more important that the present multiplicity of voluntary organisations should be co-ordinated if the importance of mental hygiene is to be adequately realised.

The Reconstruction Committee made its report in two years, but unhappily it was published at the beginning of the second world war, and so did not receive the attention which the movement had reason to expect. It was not entirely stillborn, however, because its recommendations were largely implemented under the National Health Service; and in fact it secured the complete amalgamation of three out of the four bodies referred to above, under the title of The National Association for Mental

Health. This Association has rendered continuing and valuable service since its formation, both in local activities and in the promotion of modern legislation. It has in fact established itself as one of the great voluntary organisations of the world, and works in close association with its counterparts in the United States and in many other countries. It has been an important agent in the promotion of world mental health and in the development of the World Federation.

THE UNITED STATES

The stage of development of a community plan for the care of mental disease is an excellent index of the social development of a people. In the United States, for example, the growth of mental hospitals follows a curious and interesting path parallel to that of many other advanced civilisations, and it is worth following because, in the words of Smillie 'the more intelligent and adequate the provision for the care of mental illness, the more advanced is the degree of civilisation of the community'.[1]

In colonial days the earliest hospitals in America made some provision for the care of the insane, but Virginia was the first colony to make special provision for mental illness. This was in Williamsburg and was called The Eastern State Hospital for the Insane. It was chartered in 1768. A more interesting development took place in Philadelphia in 1818, in a special institution for mental diseases established by the Quakers 'where the insane might be regarded as men and brothers'. This establishment had a remarkable parallel in Britain, where the famous York Retreat had been founded in 1792 by the Quaker citizen William Tuke. From this point onwards, the State legislators began to take an increasing interest in the care of the mentally sick. In 1821 the New York legislature appro- priated 12,500 dollars a year for fifty years to maintain the Bloomingdale Asylum, and in the same year a private institu- tion was founded in Boston by John McLain. The Hartford Retreat in Connecticut was set up in 1824, and the Massachu- setts State Insane Hospital at Worcester was built in 1830. These few cautious attempts to deal with a vast problem would not have gone at more than a snail's pace had it not been for Dorothea Dix, a great crusader, who woke the whole nation to the outstanding need for hospital care and succeeded in establishing State institutions for mental diseases throughout the entire land. The parallel with England here is John Howard.

Dorothea Dix was born in Maine in 1802. She was self-taught and became a school teacher at fourteen, and later a governess with a family in Boston. Unhappily the head of this family developed tuberculosis and several members, including the governess, were infected. In 1836 she went to England for her health and remained for a year, then she returned to Boston and took up theological training. She was assigned in 1841 as a Sunday School teacher to a class of women in the East Cambridge House of Correction. There she found, just as Howard had done in the previous century, that the insane were confined in filthy cells, neglected and maltreated. From this point she began her campaign of visits to almshouses and jails, and everywhere found the same sad story. She obtained legislative action without difficulty in Massachusetts, and then went to Rhode Island, where she received a gift for a hospital in that State. A few years later she was active in New Jersey, and finally secured funds for the great Institution for Mental Diseases at Trenton. This State held her in the highest esteem, and it was here, in this Institution, in an apartment given to her by the Trustees, that her life closed. In spite of all the difficulties, more than twenty State institutions were established as a direct result of her efforts.

EUROPE

Throughout Europe the care of persons suffering from mental disease has been one of the last medical functions assumed by the State. In the past institutions for the mentally ill, like prisons, have always been associated with coercion and restraint; and in some countries even today the location of the two institutions side by side is a grim reminder of that attitude. The modern outlook on the care of the mentally sick may be said to have emerged in Italy and France towards the end of the eighteenth century with the work of Chiarugi and Pinel in these two countries. The movement spread through Europe but unfortunately little improvement took place in actual buildings. Many countries, as they took in hand mental hospital treatment, were content to follow the worst designs, making their institutions large and gloomy. Elaborate precautions were still taken against escape, and even the interior construction of wards laid emphasis on control by force. Today the institutions used by some of the developing countries still bear scars of the old system, but there are welcome signs of a new attitude, mainly because of international progress under such bodies as the World Health Organisation and voluntary Federations. As a result of conferences and fellowships arranged by the World Health Organisation, national governments are learning more about one another, and their medical, nursing and architectural staffs are seeing for themselves what is being done in the most advanced institutions. Furthermore, many mental health authorities are finding out for themselves the sheer economic value of the humane care of the mentally sick, and particularly what can be done outside the walls of a hospital. Schemes of out-patient and home care, with trained psychiatric staff, have been widely created, but the essence of the problem is to secure and train local personnel for this work. In recent years, among many other efforts to improve conditions, comparative studies of mental hospitals in many areas of the world have been undertaken and reported upon. This is a matter of great public concern at the present time, especially when the changes introduced by the 'open door' concept of treatment have been so widely accepted.

COMMUNITY CARE AT THE PRESENT TIME

Many public health authorities are now finding out for themselves that a large proportion of successful systems of care can well be undertaken outside the walls of the hospital, whether mental or general. They have introduced schemes for out-patient and home care through the agency of clinics which have appointed trained psychiatric and auxiliary staff. A programme of this kind might develop rapidly but for the crying need for trained staff in the advancing countries; and indeed, there is no more urgent requirement at the present time than provision for training at all levels. In the first instance training has to be set on foot with the help of expert visiting teams to assist in and guide the mental health service, but as time goes on the essential needs can only be met by schemes for local training. There are therefore two stages: the first to offer fellowships to local staff to enable them to go abroad for practical training; and the second, for those who have been trained abroad to undertake teaching duties, to pass on what they have learned. A sound example of this method was provided in Taiwan. In this case the head of the department of psychiatry himself undertook a fellowship and visited many institutions in various parts of the world. On his return he set up a comprehensive training programme, arranging both theoretical and practical teaching for the local staff. By this means he introduced a plan applicable to the country as a whole.

In the developing countries the most satisfactory plan, on grounds of both economy and efficiency, would be for one country in a relatively central position to set up a joint institution for training. It should be attached to a university with a medical school so that medical students get the benefit of the teaching plan. When this has been established, it should be attractive to smaller neighbouring countries, so that teaching may be carried out at all levels. A good example of this is the Lebanon Hospital for Mental and Nervous Disorders, which has made special provision for teaching psychiatric social workers and mental nurses. In countries which are not themselves able to organise a complete system of training, the establishment of an Association for Mental Health often gives the necessary impetus towards training schemes.

Preventive Services

Up to this point we have been concerned primarily with the care of the mentally sick; but the essential aim of a health service is the prevention of disease and promotion of health. It is true, of course, in mental as in physical conditions, that a considerable amount of prevention is interwoven with treatment and after-care. It is necessary to know as much as possible about what is to be prevented, and for that reason alone clinical study and research are of vital importance. We must also know the size of the problem with which we are likely to deal, and thus statistical enquiry comes into the forefront of all preventive activities. At any rate it is now the occasion to turn to the root causes of mental disorder, and in mental health the child is the father of the man. It is now a commonplace that the origin of most of the mental troubles of adolescence and of adult life can be traced far back into childhood and even into a remoter past.

Each person enters life with a large endowment of mental and physical characteristics handed down from previous generations, and his growth as an individual is a perpetual reaction to the forces around him which we call environmental. Both hereditary and environmental factors have a profound influence on mental health, but the latter are obviously more susceptible to modification by way of preventive care. Nevertheless, the hereditary equipment is an essential part of any intelligible field of study and research. Prevention in the sense of promoting mental health is the least obtrusive and in the long run the most rewarding, of all the health measures that can be supported. The education of children, and propaganda among adults, are of great value; but there is a danger that words and pictorial methods may lack precision. In this sphere of activity preventive mental health work operates most effectively through existing agencies for health, education and child welfare, because they are understood and trusted; and in the same way the study of children is best carried out in their normal environment and in the course of their usual activities. Informality is the key to a sound approach, and preventive and promotive work cannot be successfully approached without the close co-operation of both parents and teachers. Indeed, the process of co-operation is a continuous one, beginning with the education of the older children, both boys and girls, for parenthood, and subsequently turning the full cycle through infancy, childhood and adolescence. It is in their biological setting that prevention and teaching come together to promote health.

CHILD GUIDANCE

These are the general aspects of preventive work, which apply to the normal community. The second aspect of prevention in childhood is when a disturbance of behaviour threatens or makes its first appearance. Unhappily, it is seldom possible to exert much control over the home environment, and the schools themselves vary greatly in their attitude. Difficulties and maladjustments inevitably arise, and some of these demand intervention by way of special educational treatment on account of 'emotional instability or psychological disturbance'. The overwhelming majority of maladjusted children, however, can be dealt with inside the ordinary schools, at least after preliminary guidance in a hospital psychiatric department. It is desirable that the child should be unaware as far as possible of the fact that he is singled out for any special treatment; and for this reason as well as many others there is much to be said for the association of child guidance with the normal activities of education in ordinary schools. This at once raises the important distinction between a child guidance centre, which should be part of the educational system, and a child psychiatric clinic, which should be part of the hospital system. In respect of the latter there is no value in laying stress on the idea of a special *child* clinic. Most of the treatment should in any case be directed towards the parents, and child psychiatry is best dealt with as part of an integrated psychiatric service. The children's centre, on the other hand, should work as part of the school clinic and it ought to be a focus for many of the normal health activities of the ordinary child. The school clinic makes a good centre for the work of voluntary societies concerned with children. It forms a valuable information bureau for agencies and persons interested in child welfare, as well as a place for the guidance of any child who is not developing happily in home or school environment. The centre should be able to attract a mother who is worried about her child, and it should also aim at creating a favourable attitude among the physicians working in general practice in the neighbourhood.

Much of the social effect of a child guidance centre depends on the kind of service which it is able to render both to the parent and the doctor. A general physician, let us say, is confronted with what—to him—is a difficult question of maladjusted behaviour in a child. He has heard of the existence of the centre, and decides to send mother and child there, with a letter asking for advice. In the course of time the mother returns to her physician with the report that she was kept waiting for two hours in a draughty, ill-lighted, forbidding room, without books or toys or any other means of entertainment; that she was then interviewed by someone who was evidently in a hurry, who asked a row of queer questions without explaining any reason for them. In due course the family physician receives a short note saying that the child is anxious and shows some features of depression. He knew all this already and finds the letter unhelpful; and the mother has no desire to go back to the centre. On the other hand, the mother may return with nothing but praise for the centre. She was welcomed and made to feel at home in a comfortable room where there were toys for the child and magazines for her; and there was no waiting, as an appointment had been made. The person who interviewed her took a great deal of trouble, and seemed to understand about the child, and so her mind was set at rest. A few days later the family physician received a letter stating in full the results of the interview, and giving useful guidance on how to handle the mother and treat the child.

No doubt many inappropriate patients are brought to the child guidance centre, but the sorting of children according to their needs is one of the primary functions of the staff—which ought to include a psychiatrist, an educational psychologist, and a psychiatric social worker, in addition to the school nurse and a teacher. The centre is also a valuable means of promoting child health, and parent teacher associations would find it a congenial place for their meetings and discussions. By such means the mother of the delicate child, the abnormally shy child, or the more seriously maladjusted pupil would not feel herself shut out from the normal relationships and the necessary treatment would not create a sense of isolation.

It is very difficult to assess the results of child guidance in this broad sense, and it would be hard indeed to measure the effectiveness of treatment without a prolonged and careful statistical study. In the early years of the child guidance movement some assessments were prejudiced by the fact that many children were included, who were really normal, but reacted badly to environmental difficulties. These ordinary children, whose difficulties would no doubt have cleared up in the fullness of time, recovered through simple guidance rather than psychiatric treatment, in a manner that gave pleasure to both teachers and parents. The centre received the credit it deserved, but perhaps much of the time spent would have been better occupied with the more difficult cases. It has been suggested that too much effort tends to be spent on very simple deviations which could have been equally well handled by the teachers in the ordinary school classes.The study of child psychology has already covered so much ground that there is a risk of every minor reaction being regarded as pathological. After all, growth *is* a constant process of adjustment, and in the passage through childhood to adult life there must inevitably arise disturbances of balance which will be restored by time and circumstance. The good teacher and the good parent recognise these difficulties and surmount them by patience and common-sense.

There are many contributory factors to true maladjustment; the majority arise from home and school environment as well as from individual variations in temperament. We cannot as a rule designate any one factor as 'cause' but it is commonly true that it is associated with a strong sense of insecurity, especially in relation to the other members of the family group. An actual psychological disturbance may show itself in many forms, according to the demands of the moment, but broadly speaking children who present difficulties react either by withdrawing from the struggle or by positively hostile behaviour. In schools the negative attitude is often passed over with an indulgent smile, and classified as shyness or nervousness; and solitary behaviour often passes unnoticed in the classroom, no doubt on the principle of letting sleeping dogs lie. The anti-social children, on the other hand, have an enormous nuisance value, and for this reason are usually referred to the child guidance centre. In severe and persistent cases it may be necessary to send these children to a special residential school, in the hope of avoiding the label of delinquency in adolescence. In this connection it is worth noting that a substantial number of maladjusted child-ren are physically handicapped as well, although not necessarily to a disabling extent. This points to the importance of skilled medical supervision in schools and classes for these groups. One fairly early result of faulty or delayed treatment is that the child tends to become mentally backward owing to his double handicap, and it requires a great deal of understanding to prevent this tragedy.

INTERNATIONAL CO-OPERATION

A further word should be said about mental health in the international field. Probably the first sign of co-operative effort was the International Congress of Alienists held in 1867. A much more significant advance took place with the mental hygiene movement in the United States. This was started by

Adolf Meyer, a distinguished psychiatrist, and Clifford Beers, a layman who had himself been an inmate of an asylum. These two together founded in 1909 a National Committee for Mental Hygiene. Its primary aim was to improve the treatment of mental patients and to rub out the stigma attached to mental illness. The programme of the Committee included analysis of the statistics of mental ill-health, surveys of hospitals, and the reform of legislation. Similar national associations were founded in a number of other countries following the example of this committee. In 1910 a group of Canadian and United States psychiatrists and laymen held a conference which led to the formation of the first international mental health association.

The high incidence of mental illness following the first world war gave a renewed impetus to the study of methods of prevention, and two international congresses were held between the wars on this subject. The first was in Washington in 1930 and the second in Paris in 1937. Apart from that, and the work already mentioned by the National Association for Mental Health in England, there was at that time no great emphasis on mental health in any of the bodies associated with international work. For example, in the period between the wars there were only four items listed in the bibliography of the League of Nations which referred to mental hygiene, and these dealt only with certain aspects of mental deficiency. At the same time, the International Committee for Mental Hygiene made vigorous attempts to secure the appointment of a psychiatrist on the staff of the Health Division of the League, but this was not in fact realised until the second world war was over.

A new development took place in the course of the second world war, largely because psychiatrists themselves studied preventive work with the aim of having men in jobs for which they were mentally and temperamentally suitable. The lessons learned at that time by a team of psychiatrists proved valuable later on in solving many peace-time problems. Indeed in both the American and the British Forces, psychiatrists occupied important posts in the Services, and in the first post-war International Congress on Mental Health, Dr. J. R. Rees, who had been head of the British psychiatry services, was the principal organiser. This Congress was held in London in 1948, and it

formed the World Federation for Mental Health. The first
Director General of the World Health Organisation, Dr.
Brock Chisholm, was a psychiatrist, and the first Chief of the
Mental Health Section in the Organisation was Dr. G. R. Har-
greaves, who had been one of the 'back-room boys' under
Dr. J. R. Rees during the war. When the second world war
came to an end, there was a great need for rehabilitation, both
in the physical sense and as an aspect of mental hygiene. To
begin with this work was carried out by UNRRA, and when
the technical preparatory committee for the International
Health Conference met in Paris in 1946, mental health was
already much in the minds of the delegates. Later on, when
the World Health Organisation was formed, Dr. Chisholm's
personal influence called for much greater attention to the
mental aspects of rehabilitation. Indeed the terms of the
Constitution of the World Health Organisation as finally
approved have a number of very important references to mental
health. When the first World Health Assembly took place in
Geneva priorities were allotted, and mental health took fifth
place, coming after certain urgent physical needs such as the
prevention of malaria and other epidemic diseases.

The W.H.O. Expert Committee on Mental Health met in
1949 and considered the principles on which WHO's activities
in this sphere should be based. It was obviously impossible to
lay down universally applicable rules, but the Committee made
every effort to bring into public health work the responsibility
for mental as well as physical health in the community. The
pattern was by no means simple. Even in the advanced countries there were some with highly developed therapeutic
facilities but almost no preventive services. In this way the
situation differed essentially from the task of the World Health
Organisation in relation to physical diseases, and the Committee
considered that their first activity should be to strengthen the
preventive services, integrating them wherever possible with
the other public health activities of the World Health Organisation, such as public health, nursing, and the broad issues of
education and the provision of fellowships, and also with the
work of other specialised agencies of the United Nations. As
WHO was the first international organisation to undertake the
encouragement of mental health work, it had to evolve methods

appropriate for international procedures. At first very few workers could be spared for long term assignments, and the language barrier presented a greater hindrance than in most other public health fields. The Organisation had to proceed by stimulating and planning the efforts of individual States and by adopting an approach which utilised only the newest techniques of investigation and treatment. This re-thinking of the best approach to the subject turned out to be a fascinating study and it is greatly to the credit of WHO in its earlier days that it showed such fine leadership and appreciation of the more important issues. Little time was lost on provisional arrangements and the new organisation went straight to the heart of the problem by considering each area of the world against the background of its tradition and culture.

REFERENCES

[1]SMILLIE, W. G., *History of the Public Health Service.*

Chapter 8

HOUSING

The housing of working people in the nineteenth century in response to the demands of the industrial revolution was mainly a record of failure. There are three main reasons for this. First, the population, especially of the industrial towns, was increasing rapidly. The increase itself created a pressure on accommodation in the developing industrial towns and at the same time the old cottages on farm lands were decaying and were not being replaced. This unfortunate movement led to what is known as 'jerry-building' in both the towns and villages. In England, for example, rows of dingy cottages were carelessly constructed out of old farms, barns, and even pigsties, and there was no legal control of standards. Secondly, the movement to the new industrial towns found no preparation or design on the part of the authorities, with the result that these towns grew haphazardly and so became an eyesore and a blot on the countryside. Thirdly, because there was no control by building authorities as there is today, the property owners engaged in a ruthless determination to pack as many adults into the smallest possible space and then push the children down the chinks. The result of this is still to be seen in Great Britain and Europe and many other parts of the world where industry sprang up suddenly in gaunt tenements, back-to-back houses, often without even planning of streets, and endless dingy rows of mean lanes that often lead nowhere. As so often happens, the wrong-doer had done his worst before there was any attempt by government or local authorities to control or to plan. The result was that in many towns the health officers (I use this term to include all officers concerned with planning for community health) were faced with two tasks before they could move forward—to repair the wanton damage of uncontrolled building and to redesign, often at great cost, the industrial towns and villages.

By the beginning of the twentieth century in England two

conclusions about housing had been reluctantly accepted: the first that it was no longer possible for private enterprise to build houses for workers alone and let houses at an economic rent, and secondly, that the state must take over some respons- ibility, not only for building houses but also for planning, design and the establishment of standards. This urgent issue was dealt with by legislation* but the main problem of rebuilding was postponed for another twenty years because of the great increase in public transport through the development of subways, street cars and buses. These advances suddenly extended the land suitable for low rent housing.

Similar patterns were followed in other countries, and unhappily are being adopted today in many of those which stand on the threshold of industrial development. Standards vary enormously and have done so up and down through many generations. Unfortunately, in the face of rising costs, there is always the risk that standards of housing will be lowered. Shakespeare put the matter in a nutshell:

'When we mean to build,
We first survey the plot, then draw the model;
And when we see the figure of the house,
Then must we rate the cost of the erection;
Which, if we find outweighs ability,
What do we then but draw anew the model
In fewer offices, or at least desist
To build at all?'
And the last state is worse than the first:
'Like one that draws the model of a house
Beyond his power to build it; who, half through,
Gives o'er and leaves his part-created cost
A naked subject to the weeping clouds,
And waste for churlish Winter's tyranny.'
(King Henry IV, Part II, Act 1, Scene 3)

During the industrial revolution, as we have seen, there were no standards at all. Indeed there must be some variation between the rural cottages on the one hand and the town housing on the other; some variation between the shack in Brazil and a cottage in Sweden. One cannot expect a shack to have all the conveniences of modern life, nor indeed the country cottage—a piped water supply, a water-carriage

*E.g. The Housing of the Working Classes Act of 1890.

H

system of sewage disposal, gas and electric light, and the frequent collection of refuse. Yet there must be for all dwellings, whether in Europe or Africa or any other continent, some minimum requirement of comfort, domestic convenience, space, light and air. Florence Nightingale set down these requirements many years ago:

There are five essential points in securing the health of houses:—

1. Pure air
2. Pure water
3. Efficient drainage
4. Cleanliness
5. Light.

The tragedy of the situation is that we do not learn from history. As recently as 1958 the following description was written of a 'new town' in Africa:

This village was originally a hamlet too small to be shown on the maps of the area, but today it is a rapidly growing settlement. Houses of the poorest type are being erected on every piece of open land, and the roofs of many touch those of the adjoining buildings. Additional rooms are continually being added to existing houses as the demand for accommodation increases. The ceiling height of many of these does not exceed four feet at the external wall. There are usually six to eight occupants to each room.

The only water supply is provided by the nearby swamp. There are no latrines whatsoever, and the whole area for some distance round the village is fouled by human excrement. Everyone has money to purchase canned provisions, and there are empty food tins in quantity lying around every house. These, together with the excrement, are giving rise to massive fly-breeding.

Instances of this could be multiplied indefinitely, not only in the developing countries, which might learn by following the best examples, but also in the fully industrial countries such as Britain and the United States, where sordid building is still all too common and the slum is a persistent companion. In Great Britain, for example, within the last decade there were fourteen million dwellings and of these nearly six million were over sixty-five years old. Many of these are dilapidated, but the great bulk of them are only too substantial, though wretchedly lacking in modern amenities. The health officer of a large borough reported that 75 per cent of the houses in his area had no baths. If these old houses continue to be left as they so often were in Brooklyn, London or Rio de Janeiro, they will deteriorate beyond remedy and not infrequently they suffer a still worse fate of being divided up into small apartments, each one holding a family but none sufficient to hold a single person.

In considering the subject of building and then planning at the international level, we are faced with a number of difficulties. The first is that nature herself conspires against definition, because climate and geography so greatly alter the needs or indeed the maximum that can be expected in any one place. There is little in common between Northern Finland and Sierra Leone, or between the rain-soaked tropics and the hot desert, even on the same continent. In fact we are dealing with at least two, and probably three, worlds of natural conditions alone, without reference to man. Unhappily, we have several worlds of mankind, with hardly anything in common with regard to social and economic conditions—and even education. How is it possible to devise standards which can be applied intelligently to a modern American, Scandinavian, or British city and at the same time to the following, on which a colleague of mine has recently reported? We are dealing briefly with an eastern city which has a university and a medical school. It is the centre of a state of over sixty million people. Here are the chill facts:

The literacy rate is 10.8%, and of these 80% were only just literate. The local people, although intelligent and religious, are superstitious, uneducated and deeply fatalistic . . . in 1959 a member of the department conducted a sample survey in the area surrounding the health centre, covering a population of 5,313. It revealed that 98% of the houses had no latrines, and that 88% of the families drew water from open, shallow wells, all of which showed evidence of recent or past pollution of animal and vegetable origin. The birth rate was 40 per thousand, and the death rate 39. The high death rate was due mainly to smallpox and tuberculosis, each of which was responsible for 17.6% of the total deaths; and to the infant mortality rate of 189 per thousand.

At this moment we deserve a contrast or we shall collapse. My first visit to Finland was just after their war, at the time when the Russians had made peace. One of the most interesting visits I was privileged to make was to the brilliant architect,

Alvar Aalto. Among other things we discussed the restoration of the Arctic villages which had been destroyed by the retiring soldiers. It will be remembered that the building season in that country is very short, and that it is death to be without a habitation. Accordingly, I asked Aalto what he planned to do, as he was the Government's official adviser. He replied simply:

The prime needs of the people are shelter, warmth and water. So we shall put up houses in their barest simplicity, with only the skeleton of a second floor, but with full protective insulation of roof, walls and floor. In what will be the living room we shall instal an efficient type of Finnish stove to burn wood; and finally we shall lay a single water pipe to each home, rising through the floor from deep underground, below the extreme freezing level. That is all. But in preparation for winter work indoors we shall provide for each village a depot where they can obtain at a low cost such materials as wood for flooring, kitchen sinks, hot water tanks, and so on. During the long months of darkness the village folk will take some training and help to build up the features that turn a shelter into a home.

One more illustration will suffice—this time in Algeria:

This is a model in miniature of the unstable demographic situation found in many African countries today. The more than nine million Moslem population far outnumbers the one and a half million of European origin ... In essence, two distinct Algerias exist today. They differ markedly in education, religion, living levels, etc. One is essentially urban-European, and the other is rural. The Moslems, who are predominantly agricultural, exist at a semi-starvation level in a land almost barren. Nine out of ten Moslems are illiterate, unable to read or write in either Arabic or French. In contrast, the European colonists are largely city-dwellers whose levels of living, health, and education are not much different from those of the French living in Metropolitan France.

(Population Profile : April 14, 1961, Washington 5, D.C.)

So this is where we stand, and one must realise that it would make nonsense to prescribe a single housing standard for these extremes. Yet there are some essentials for both worlds. My personal experience in house visiting and inspection has been largely in Europe and Northern America, and I have seen and studied slum conditions as far apart as Athens, Glasgow, Lisbon, New York, Chicago and San Francisco. This is all very well, but what I am most anxious to find is the beginning of a definition that would even give some details, if not fundamentals. My colleague, George Macdonald,* who has an immense knowledge of tropical conditions, suggests that the essential requirements of a house in relation to health are that it should provide:

1. Shelter from the rain, wind, and extremes of climate. It should be of such a construction that, with or without appliances, it is reasonably possible to maintain it in a comfortable climatic environment. This could be defined in terms of a range of effective temperature or equivalent temperature.

2. The essential facilities for clean living and particularly:
   (a) readily accessible potable water;
   (b) provision for the safe storage and preparation of food; and
   (c) provision for the safe disposal of excreta and wastes.

3. The background necessary to its care by the occupants, in particular:
   (a) it should be free from sources of avoidable dirt, whether internal, as by smoking chimneys, structural, as in unpainted or otherwise fissured walls, or external, as by waterlogged or fouled surroundings;
   (b) all parts of living space should be reasonably accessible for cleaning;
   (c) it should be free from dilapidation and damp;
   (d) provision should be made, separately from living rooms, for the storage of bulky material, such as firewood, necessary to its maintenance;
   (e) adequate light and ventilation.

4. The minimum possible shelter for noxious pests.

5. The environment necessary for a healthy family life, in accordance with the special and cultural requirements of the community concerned.

Now here, as Macdonald points out, is a series of requirements which could be applied with equal validity to a simple rural habitation in the tropics and to a town house in a temperate country. And he wisely adds that the standards applicable to a country such as Great Britain are not necessarily applicable to, *or even acceptable to,* the peoples of other countries.

There are many examples of careful analysis of the principles of healthful housing and in the United States the standard work on the subject was produced by a Committee on the

*M.D., D.T.M., F.R.C.P., London School of Hygiene and Tropical Medicine.

Hygiene of Housing (American Public Health Association) under the Chairmanship of C.-E.A. Winslow, Dr. P. H.). This work was produced in 1941 and contained in the appendix a brief note about the 'Basic Principles of Healthful Housing'.

In Great Britain the Ministry of Health* has produced several valuable memoranda showing the progressive acceptance of clearer requirements in housing, and it is of great interest to follow the standards as they are raised from one issue to another in response to informed opinion.

Apart from sporadic efforts in some advanced countries, there has been little concerted attempt to improve the housing of workers until the nineteenth century. Great cities have arisen in the past with magnificent buildings, but the control of environment with the direct aim of improving the people's health is a recent development. Great credit is due to some of the pioneers like John Howard, who built a village to replace the ill-housed rural workers on his own estate; and to Robert Owen, who made the fine experiment of creating a new industrial town which brought together a healthy residential environment and equally sound conditions in the factories themselves.

As the nineteenth century proceeded, a number of men of social imagination put forward plans for local and national consideration of the housing problem, but it was Edwin Chadwick's report on the *Sanitary Conditions of the Labouring Population of Great Britain,* produced as an official document in 1842, that really shocked people of goodwill and set housing activities in motion. A few years later in 1850, Lemuel Shattuck in Boston, Massachusetts, wrote a brilliant *Report of the Sanitary Commission of Massachusetts.* He went further than Chadwick in recognising the need for planning as well as sanitary construction.

In England, the creation of voluntary 'Health of Towns Associations' did much to promote public interest in the housing conditions of the working poor, but it was not until the middle of the century that the great social reformer, Lord Shaftesbury, was able to introduce two Acts of Parliament designed to meet the worst of the situation. Throughout the century, as we have seen, housing development proceeded a

* Now 'Housing and Local Government'.

little erratically but the closing years of the nineteenth century brought together many interests and Parliament was really stirred in consequence of reports of the Royal Sanitary Commission in 1869 and many other detailed accounts of conditions, especially from the larger cities. It is noteworthy, however, that there was no town planning act, even in name, until shortly before the first world war, when a very weak statute of 1909 obtained recognition for planning as a vital need in the development of towns.

In the international field little attention was given to the problems of housing until after the first world war. In 1922 the International Labour Office made a start with the problems of urban and rural housing with special reference to providing for the workers' health and well-being. In 1931 the Health Organisation of the League of Nations undertook an important series of studies of rural housing. This occupied a considerable proportion of its time and interest until three years later the Bureau of the Health Committee, acting upon a resolution adopted at the Assembly of 1934, established a Housing Commission. This Commission supported reviews of housing conditions in seven European countries and proceeded in a more general way to extend the study to some of the most important aspects of the hygiene of housing and of national urban and rural planning. In addition to these activities, the Commission also stimulated the formation of national committees of housing and health in several countries to co-operate with the main programme of the Commission. Unfortunately the onset of world war II brought these activities to an end, but it was not long before interest was renewed. When delegates to the International Health Conference, which was held in 1946, came to study the important health problems which the World Health Organisation should face, they made a special point in its draft constitution of including the importance of housing and other aspects of environmental hygiene. Indeed, the first World Health Assembly gave high priority to environmental sanitation, and suggested that future programmes should include housing and town planning. These actions indicate clearly that the World Health Organisation recognised the importance of the relationship between housing and the state of health and well-being of a population.

At the international level several governmental agencies have shown an increasing interest in the problems of housing and health. The United Nations Bureau of Social Affairs— Housing, Building and Planning Branch—is concerned with many problems of housing at the international level and has conducted seminars to give advice appropriate to many different geographic areas. The International Labour Organisation has devoted a great deal of time to the study of housing accommodation of workers under different conditions and has examined especially new industries in the developing countries. The Economic Commissions of the United Nations have also created special housing units which have been active in assisting governments in studying ways and means of solving their housing problems, with special emphasis on the economic, financial, administrative and statistical aspects.

In addition to this, the Food and Agricultural Organisation has in recent years placed a growing emphasis on subjects related to housing. One of the more important of these covers research studies on the development and use of forest products in building. There has also been a significant development of housing centres, and within the United Nations, inter-Agency working groups on Housing and Related Community Facilities were created in 1956. The whole subject of research in housing has in fact received greatly increased attention and it is significant that the studies have become progressively wider in their relation to health, with emphasis on a team approach and greater co-ordination between the various technical groups, e.g. engineers and public health officers.

In general, it would seem that rapid industrial development without proper town planning inevitably leads to public health risks, both personal and environmental. In the case of the former, one must include the increased liability to infection, especially among children, and more extensive complications of the common diseases of childhood.

It has been said that we build the homes of yesterday for the people of tomorrow. In her book 'Nation and Family'[1] Alva Myrdal observes that 'the housing supply is the least flexible of all major items involved in social change' and she adds that the lag in housing often serves as one of the most important factors in retarding both the rise in the standard of living and the adjustment of family life to the changing composition and changing work of the average family. 'Other consumption habits', she says, 'will react more quickly to new movements. We may learn to eat foods rich in vitamins and to wear suitable clothing, but in our most important modes of living we shall continue to be limited by the conceptions of yesterday because the very houses determine so much of our everyday life'.

Even in the fully advanced countries housing development has undoubtedly lagged far behind any other social changes and a large proportion of the population must inevitably live in dwellings inherited from an older generation. We are in fact always dragging our feet behind, replanning and rebuilding for modern conditions.

In environmental services the risk of a breakdown in public health services such as overtaxing the water and drainage systems, failing in measures of food protection, cleaning of streets and public buildings, and general environmental services is greatly increased by lack of planning. In some of the developing regions of the world the problem arises of the retention of the 'old city' of narrow, winding streets and densely packed buildings. There is much to be said for retaining old buildings if they have historical associations or possess intrinsic beauty. At the same time the old town must be a part of the total planning scheme, carefully designed to prevent the crowding in of housing or industrial buildings. It may, of course, preserve its traditional artisan crafts, its commercial activities such as bazaars, and some of its old buildings can be converted into appropriate new uses.

When towns grow at great speed, however, one has to consider and balance the advantages of preservation against threats to human welfare. On the one hand there is a real danger of building cheap and shoddy dwellings wherever there happens to be a space, without regard to the welfare of the tenants or of the city as a whole. The second danger, which must be guarded against even more, is gross overcrowding. What happens is that old houses and tenements which were suitable for families half a century ago are redesigned with the object of cramming as many families as possible into inferior accommodation. Then it often happens that these older buildings do not provide enough, and the authorities permit a zone of huts or shacks to spread like an infection, without any social organisation. Lastly, if the land on the outskirts has to be used, it is often of inferior quality, such as a half-filled swamp, or even an old refuse dump left by the original builders because it was unsuitable.

The distressing problem is: how are the health functions to be carried out? The first answer, and in many respects the most vital, is that cheap housing without proper planning is the most expensive of all forms of building. The reason for this is obvious, because water supplies and drainage have to be put in at great cost sooner or later if they have been omitted in the first instance. Environmental services grow best when they are firmly rooted in community life and are planned along with other forms of living. In new towns as well as in villages, they ought to be an essential part of the community programme, and the enthusiasm of the inhabitants is the only guarantee of continuing success.

The second answer is that the public health services cannot be set moving in isolation; they must be associated with other community activities such as road-making, land drainage, and every form of co-operation with neighbouring communities.

The third point is—and I must lay great stress on it— that no housing and town planning activity has any hope of success without the help of *law* as a preventive measure. We are apt to think of law as mainly restrictive and penal, but this is quite a wrong conception when it comes to doing things right *in the first instance*, and in that all technical and lay people need the guidance of legislation—basic rules of conduct.

Before proceeding further, we come to this: that no permanent advance can be expected in the absence of an educated and understanding community: educated, that is, to appreciate the benefits of a sound, practical health programme which is well within the range of their everyday vision.

The features of bad housing conditions have not substantially changed since the beginning of state intervention. The emphasis has been altered in some degree but the essential factors are the same.

POVERTY

It has been shown again and again that there is a close relation between economic status and the number of persons per room, but here you at once bring in the confusing element of overcrowding. There is no doubt, however, that poverty drives families into lower housing conditions and these in turn intensify the ill effects on the family and form a kind of vicious circle of poverty, ill-housing and sickness.

OCCUPATION

In the nineteenth century during the era of great industrial progress unhealthy occupations were all too common. We know a great deal about the boy chimney sweeps and the conditions of the miners and knife-grinders, but there was in addition an enormous amount of less published sickness in sweated industries and particularly in the small workshops and the homes where women and children had to carry out jobs under exceedingly unfavourable conditions. Unhealthy occupations and bad housing conditions were interlocked because of the deliberate slum building in the industrial towns of the nineteenth century. In recent years fortunately a great deal has been done to eliminate positively unhealthy jobs where there is a known hazard to health, but bad housing and wretched occupations still conspire together.

MEDICAL CARE

In one respect, in England at any rate, bad housing conditions are associated with good medical care. What we mean is that a great deal of public money is being spent not only on the National Health Service but also on the preventive and social services among the lower income groups. Those who live in slums have pretty good opportunities for attending hospitals and clinics and of obtaining extra supplies of milk and special foods. In this sense it could be argued that the preventive services are to some extent salvage, because they are spending time, effort and public money in dealing with conditions that could be eliminated by better housing. In many other countries, such as the United States, where they have no National Health Service, it has been shown that the lower income groups have more sickness and less medical and dental care than the more prosperous.

PERSONAL FACTORS IN THE FAMILIES

There is no doubt that slum areas have more than their share of the dull-witted and the ignorant and this is only to be expected. We may ask ourselves whether indifferent parents readily get into a poor environment and whether the defects we find in their children are due to the environment or to parental neglect. I remember in a study of the distribution of enlarged tonsils and adenoids we found no great difference in incidence at the various economic levels but it was evident that treatment was undertaken earlier and more frequently in the upper groups, and that serious complications, like otitis media, were much more common in the lower groups.

SICKNESS

Chronic sickness is a notorious cause of loss of earning power and in countries where there is little provision against sickness and unemployment the weaker are driven down readily to the worst housing conditions.

INFECTIOUS DISEASE

When we turn to the common infections it is clear that there is a strong association with overcrowding but not necessarily with other bad housing conditions. I think the most that can be said apart from overcrowding is that it is much more difficult to nurse a sick child where the housing is bad and therefore there is an increased tendency to secondary infections, especially in such diseases as measles and scarlet fever. Again, isolation of a sick person becomes virtually impossible and the whole household is in league against recovery.

The various disorders lumped together under the heading of rheumatism are commonly believed to be associated with damp houses. I have never found any real success in attempts to prove the relationship—indeed the most recent studies rather tend the other way (Stevenson and Cheeseman). We do recognise that a cold, damp climate provokes a tendency to rheumatism and transfer to a hot, dry area gives temporary relief.

OVERCROWDING

This is by far the most important element of bad housing. In 1930 we used to think, in our innocence, that if we could destroy enough slums and house the same people in better areas we should have solved the housing problem. We now realise rather sadly that we started at the wrong end: we should have tried first of all to reduce overcrowding and then we could have set about slum clearance more systematically with at least a sufficient number of roofs to cover the heads of most families. We may not have much exact information about ill effects of bad housing but there is no doubt whatever about overcrowding. The Registrar-General has repeatedly shown that the death rate of young children from the main causes of death in the big cities is more closely related to the proportion of people living in overcrowded conditions than with climate or geographical situations. Indeed the mortality in overcrowded areas is about three times as great in young children.

The burden of the common infectious diseases also falls very heavily on young children in tenements and other overcrowded areas. This is not because of an increase in the number affected; it is the complications such as bronchitis and pneumonia that take the heaviest toll. Density of child population is a most important factor; for example in measles, overcrowding produces its disastrous effect by causing an early age of attack and so leading to high mortality and the more frequent respiratory complications. Whooping cough, which is the most serious of all infections of childhood, is specially liable to attack those who are already weak and so it finds easy victims in bad housing conditions and most particularly where there is added overcrowding.

The death rate, however, represents only a fraction of the harm done; there is a good deal of evidence that overcrowding as such, that is the huddling together of people in a confined space, produces bad effects on health, yet it is hard to produce exact proof, especially if we are not careful to study the conditions under which families are actually living. The average number of persons per room is often an unsure guide. In one London borough, for example, we have the figure of 0·80, which is better than that of the country as a whole, and very much better than that of a neighbouring borough, with 1·01. All the same, the amount of overcrowding is far greater in fact in this London borough among the really overcrowded, because 12·6 per cent of the families are living at densities of more than two persons per room, compared with 10·2 per cent in the neighbouring borough, and 6·9 per cent in the country as a whole.

Again, we find great differences in the habits of people. In countries where central heating is the rule, the family is commonly pretty well distributed unless the house is very small indeed, but in Great Britain, where we are often dependent on a single fire in the living room and no heating elsewhere, parents and children tend to be huddled together in one room to get some warmth in winter. It is interesting, for example, to compare urban dwellings in Britain with those in Sweden. Our houses are comparatively spacious but in Sweden it is not uncommon to have the rooms very small indeed; with central heating, however, one would expect the Swedish family to distribute itself in the best possible way throughout the house. We huddle our families together because of lack of warmth, but in Sweden it is not uncommon for the same crowding to take place in one small room for the sake of the prestige of having one elegant apartment reserved for visitors. Again we in our larger cities, like Glasgow, effectively combine overcrowding with slum conditions; the Swedish people do not tolerate slums and the Swedish housewife will probably have to be scolded for too much cleaning and polishing rather than too little.

We must not think of overcrowding in terms of readily diagnosable disease. The greater trouble lies on the mental side—the difficulty of living together in overcrowded conditions. Take, for example, lack of sleep. In an overcrowded dwelling persons of different ages ought to have different times for going to bed. The activities of the adult encroach on the rest that the children need. The play space of small children becomes hopelessly cramped and there is constant repression because a good housewife's ambition to keep order is always in conflict with every child's proper demand for freedom and space for its play. The same difficulty is intensified when children reach school age and want space for quiet and study. The growing child tends to lose his individuality in a crowded home. For adolescents the loss is even greater because of lack of privacy and the impossibility of bringing in their young friends.

Everything that happens in a crowded home has to be experienced by everybody.

TUBERCULOSIS

When we come to study some of the more important causes of disability such as tuberculosis and acute rheumatism, we are at once struck by the effects of overcrowding. The most interesting studies have been made by Lilli Stein in Edinburgh and Glasgow. She made a careful analysis of small, well-defined localities instead of the larger areas, and chose comparable groups with the common characteristics of overcrowding and similar classification of tenants. From her studies she found a strong relationship between the incidence and death rate of respiratory tuberculosis and true overcrowding in the home. Another obvious effect in respiratory tuberculosis is the impossibility of properly isolating the patient, and this applies to rural areas just as much as to urban. It has been shown repeatedly that children in households containing an adult suffering from tuberculosis of the lung are subject to a much higher death rate from tuberculosis than other children of their age group. In Newcastle-upon-Tyne, for example, Miller, in 1947, showed that from June 1941 to December 1945 his team had examined 520 children under the age of five years; 369 had been contacts of pulmonary tuberculosis and 151 of other types of the disease. At the first examination 142 of the 369 contacts were tuberculin-positive; of 151 contacts of other types of tuberculosis 12 were positive. The mortality from tuberculosis in the 369 children in contact with pulmonary tuberculosis was 5 per cent to December 1945. In children under the age of five years, 30 per cent of the morbidity and 30 per cent of the total mortality from tuberculosis occurred in a small group at special risk.

Some years ago we heard a lecturer say we must get rid of the slum mentality before we moved the slum families into new houses. I once heard a member of the Education Committee say in public that children must learn to keep their hands and their faces clean and then they would be provided with soap and towels.

In visiting houses, we may sometimes wonder what tests to employ to decide between a bad house and a bad tenant. The character and the capacity of the tenant is a vital element in slum making. It is not always easy to determine where the fault lies as between the house and its management. Here are one or two useful tests, however, that can be borne in mind:

1. Are the bedclothes and the children's clothes in good repair? The test does not require them to be new, of good material, or even thoroughly clean.

2. Is there any filth in the house that must necessarily have accumulated over several days? The mere fact that there is rubbish lying about at the time of a visit is no test of management.

3. Is there some attempt at order in the food store, with protection of materials (like milk) that are easily contaminated? The test does not require the food store to be tidy at the time of inspection, or even spotlessly clean. The experienced investigator soon learns what standards ought to be accepted as a minimum.

If the housewife does not pass these three simple tests, then further investigation is necessary, even in a dilapidated dwelling. There are many possible answers:

1. The woman, although healthy, may be quite unable to cope with the burden of her work. The usual causes for this are that she has a large family, that she has to go out to work, that there is a sick, defective or infirm member of the family requiring more or less constant attention.

2. The housewife is ill, or has some physical disability which interferes with her work. Rheumatism and other crippling conditions and defective eyesight are common causes.

3. The woman, although physically healthy, is mentally unable to cope with the domestic situation. Mental deficiency or severe educational backwardness in one or other of the parents is the main cause, and is believed to account for about fifty per cent of all 'undesirable tenants'. The most difficult type is the 'borderline', not certifiable as mentally defective, yet socially incompetent.

4. The tenants who do not care form a small but hard core of the undesirables. They neglect their homes and their children, and they are generally not merely socially incompetent but positively anti-social. They are the incorrigible slum-makers, the lees of humanity. The causes are various: the results of a

broken home or other reason depriving them of a family life
of their own; delinquency, drink, vice, or the deliberate choice
of a life of crime. We may regard them as carriers of social
disease, or what we will, but at any rate there they are.

REFERENCE

[1]MYRDAL, ALVA (1941): *Nation and Family,* New York, Harper Brothers.

I

Chapter 9

VOLUNTARY SERVICE

The voluntary health agency as we know it in many countries today is a modern organisation which started out to furnish health services of a kind which had not previously been given. It was a pioneer in putting to use for the common welfare new facts or new concepts about health and disease. While in total capacity the voluntary health movements had their fullest flowering in the United States, there are other countries, notably the Netherlands, which practically depend for their official health services on voluntary work supported by the Government. In the United States, many of the organisations, such as the Henry Street Settlement and the Association for Improving the Condition of the Poor, developed both nursing and clinical services and were in fact services rather than movements. The funds raised by voluntary health societies in total amounted to something like six million dollars annually. This includes the work of the Red Cross and certain philanthropic organisations for the promotion of health.

The National Tuberculosis Association is the oldest agency in the United States rendering actual services. Only half a century ago tuberculosis was the chief single cause of death and produced an enormous amount of chronic illness and disability among its victims. At that time there was no known cure. To avoid being stigmatised, individuals and families with tuberculous members made every effort to conceal the presence of the disease. In 1882, when Koch discovered the tubercle bacillus, the concept of tuberculosis as an infection was finally established. More than ten years elapsed, however, between the discovery of the bacillus and the beginning of the first organised campaign for treatment and cure. Meanwhile, the implications for community action had been recognised in Great Britain, France and several other European countries. Robert W. Philip (1857-1939) saw that 'if the community as such was to benefit practically by the discovery, there appeared to be need of centralised effort in order to ascertain the extent of tuberculosis in a district, and to devise means for its limitation and prevention.' The result was the opening, in 1887, of the Edinburgh Victoria Dispensary for Consumption—the first tuberculosis dispensary in the world. Philip's programme also included home visiting, health education and an occupational farm colony for patients. This pioneer work was followed in 1898 by the organisation of the National Association for the Prevention of Consumption and other forms of Tuberculosis. Its objects were similar to those in the United States.

On the continent of Europe the same ideas were developed independently. A French League Against Tuberculosis was founded in 1891 by Armingaud of Bordeaux. In June of the same year the National League for the Campaign against Tuberculosis was organised in Denmark, and in 1899 Calmette, who introduced BCG vaccine, conceived the idea of tuberculosis clinics for prevention, education and ambulatory treatment. In 1901, he and his associates opened the first dispensary in Lille, and by the end of 1905 there were no less than 62 of these establishments in France. Similar movements took place gradually in Germany and other countries of Europe. In the United States, as early as 1889, a report on community action against tuberculosis had been drawn up by Herman M. Biggs, J. Mitchell Prudden and H. P. Loomis. They recommended that the Department of Health itself should keep track of the disease in New York City, and be responsible for public education. Finally, in 1894, the Department began to require reporting of the cases of tuberculosis by institutions, and three years later this was extended to physicians. Similar efforts were made in other parts of the United States, especially in Baltimore and Philadelphia. It would be fair to say that tuberculosis was the disease in which the first public health programme for prevention and health education was introduced. The Pensylvania Society for the Prevention of Tuberculosis, formed in 1892, was the pioneer association. This was the first body to endeavour to marshal the forces of the community by combining lay and professional membership, and its pattern has been widely followed up to the present time. The objective of the Society was to be achieved:

1. By promulgating the doctrine of the contagiousness of the disease.

2. By instructing the public in practical methods of avoidance and prevention.

3. By visiting the consumptive poor and supplying them with the necessary materials with which to protect themselves against the disease, and instructing them in their use.

4. By furnishing the consumptive poor with hospital treatment.

5. By co-operating with Boards of Health in such measures as they may adopt for the prevention of the disease.

6. By advocating the enactment of appropriate laws for the prevention of the disease.

7. By such other methods as the Society may from time to time adopt.

So far we have been considering, very briefly, the action of voluntary bodies in the attempt to hold back the great scourges of mankind, of which tuberculosis has been chosen as an example. One of the difficulties that has been shown, again and again, in discussions on quarantine is the failure to achieve concerted action, due to natural suspicion of one nation towards another, and to the restrictions that might be imposed on merchants and traders. Fortunately, there is another means of securing a better understanding between peoples. The principles of voluntary co-operation with Governments were demonstrated by the Rockefeller Foundation in connection with the extension of their great hookworm campaign, and these have retained their force up to the present time. The basis of action, as the Rockefeller Health Board stated, was that it should 'act as a partner but not as a patron'. That is to say, the Foundation furnished technical leadership and a graduated portion of the cost of the enterprise, but the country itself was also required to assist and contribute financially; the project was always an integral part of the machinery of Government. One of the secrets of the subsequent success of the grants made and the plans undertaken by the Foundation was that it required local participation—that is of the Government and the community.

It is noteworthy that in the early days of the hookworm campaign, Wycliffe Rose and his colleagues were accustomed to speak of the *eradication* of the disease. At a later date, this expression was to become more significant in the greater struggle against malaria. For a variety of reasons, hookworm never was eradicated, but it was confined within a manageable compass and has become, like typhoid and smallpox, a controllable disease. In some ways, this was a more important conception: that the strategy against hookworm was a new advance in preventive medicine—a demonstration in disease control which could readily be understood and accepted by a community.

This kind of combination of ideas led Rose to his next great effort. He began to realise that although remarkable advances had been made in scientific studies of malaria, it was still responsible for more sickness and death than all other diseases. As early as 1915, he began a series of experimental projects with the object of finding out how to control malaria, and whether this could be done at a reasonable cost, within the means of an average community. Once he had satisfied himself that simple measures could sharply reduce the incidence of the disease, he began to dream of the application of preventive measures on a far wider scale. His mind turned to the strategy against hookworm which had already proved its worth— demonstration and education. Five years of work in the United States on an ever widening range led him to put forward a bold scheme with the world as his parish. In 1916, when a marked increase in malaria occurred in the South of France, the International Health Board accepted a request from the French Government to lead a campaign. This was only a demonstration. What Rose had in mind was the creation among States and Nations of some permanent machinery through which the whole field of public health could be surveyed and staffs created to deal in advance with threats to health. In other words, he hoped that the International Board would leave behind it, wherever it rendered service, a determination to set up machinery and staff for a modern health department. Rose felt strongly that unless a stable health department and service were instituted by the local health authority, the work of a private agency would be constantly defeated by subsequent neglect. This concept of 'pump priming' was applied to hundreds of authorities and before long it had been projected like a rocket around the world.

Sydney Smith once wrote, 'It is important that there should be as many *understandings* in the world as possible', and he concluded his vivid essay in the year 1810, with this comment:

'The instruction of women improves the stock of national talents and employs more minds for the instruction and amusement of the world. . . . The education of women favours public morals; it provides for every season of life, as well as for the brightest and the best; and leaves a woman when she is stricken by the hand of time, not as she is now, destitute of everything and neglected by all; but with the full power and the spendid attractions of knowledge.'

One of the most striking movements in Great Britain was the Women's Voluntary Service. It all began in 1938, when war with Germany seemed imminent. The Home Secretary, at that time Sir Samuel Hoare, approached Lady Reading, with a view to recruiting women to help in work associated with Air Raid Precautions. The response was remarkably good. The movement began with a membership of 5, and by the end of the year it was 300,000. The first task of these women was to prepare for evacuation. This was done in conjunction with the Local Authorities and a Billeting Survey was made.

When Germany invaded Poland in 1939, this scheme was put into operation with remarkable speed. In three days one-and-a-quarter million children with their mothers were evacuated from the big cities to safe areas in the country. There was a considerable lull before any adverse action was taken, with the result that many children were returned to their homes, but in May 1940 the evacuation really began, and refugees poured into the country.

The W.V.S. had innumerable tasks to do, and they had to learn by experience, in all weathers, in blackouts and in raids. It says a great deal for the Organisation of W.V.S. that in this nightmare of confusion, individuals received consideration and assistance. This included food and clothing, and many other kinds of assistance; the collection of salvage, and every conceivable type of human help, both for protection of those who were threatened and for hospital care of the injured.

The provision of Rest Centres was one of the important services throughout the country, as these Centres offered help of every kind, including food and clothing to those who were in distress. This included provision for the homeless, and above all the organisation of a service which completely prevented chaos.

All the workers had to be provided for, as well as the sufferers, and in every area food, transport and clothing needs were quickly met. All sorts of canteens were provided. Libraries were brought into use and newspapers sent by land and sea.

In addition to universal care for citizens who belonged to Britain, provision had to be made on the same scale for American troops as well as for mine-sweepers and small naval craft.

When the War came to an end, these innumerable activities had to be curtailed. This appeared to reduce the need for the W.V.S., but so much had to be done in the way of clearance that the work of the W.V.S. was hardly reduced. Its members had to help families to settle down, and much in the way of confusion had to be sorted out. British and allied prisoners-of-war, for example, began to return from Germany; the W.V.S. helped to receive them at the airfields, and dispersal camps were organised with great speed.

Towards the end of 1943, the troop welfare services were extended to combat zones abroad, and a similar high standard of service was given all over the combat area. The demand for the W.V.S. extended so far as Korea, and indeed became world wide.

The activities of the W.V.S. were far from concluded; the winters were severe, and there would have been much suffering especially among the elderly people if there had not been visits to old people, and help of every kind as part of the assistance given. Residential clubs were provided by the generosity of private donors, and help was given until houses could be secured.

The help provided by the W.V.S. has maintained its efficiency. This includes hospital care services in co-operation with the existing societies, and especially aid to elderly people who are not actually ill but who would benefit by visits to relatives and meals to the sick. Arrangements have also been made to give holidays to children in need of a change to fresh air. Handicapped people are also provided for in connection with schools and hospitals, and also in their own homes.

These are only a fraction of the services rendered by the

W.V.S. in peace-time, and it is clear that this organised voluntary service of women has come to stay.

Another example of voluntary activity associated with philanthropic motive amounted to the desire by one's personal action to make life better for others. Early in the nineteenth century, both in England and in America, this motive found expression chiefly in works of charity and moral uplift. It was the age of religious tracts—and of laissez-faire. The mid-century passed on the motive to schemes of 'relief' and doles, and was represented by the appointment of women on Poor Law Boards. As time went on, the philanthropic motive began to lose its head, and all kinds of abuses crept in, especially the ill-usage of hospitals, and a sinister trading in multiple charities. It was for this reason that the Charity Organisation Society was created, and there is no doubt that it did splendid work at a critical period.

In the United States the old Poor Law of England was carried across the ocean, and so governmental aid came before voluntary action. In 1863, however, the Massachusetts Board of Charities was formed as a commission of citizens, with a paid secretary; and within ten years there were Boards in nine States. This was the first step in the creation of a new profession —the social worker. The next move took place in Philadelphia with the formation in 1879 of the 'Society for Organising Charity', which had the double aim of organising existing charities into a compact whole, and of creating a new kind of service of trained workers in the social field. The admitted success of these bodies in both countries showed the crying need for them, as local government bodies had difficulty in incorporating voluntary workers. But in many ways the opposition between governmental assistance and the C.O.S. was unfortunate, especially in the later stages, when it became obvious in times of war and depression that purely voluntary effort was not enough. It may well be that the second function of the Charity Organisation Society was the more vital to public welfare—the drawing out of men and women of goodwill to serve as leaders in social work.

There are many voluntary motives for State action today. In the United Kingdom, as people stand and watch the vast changes in health and social work that have characterised the middle of the twentieth century, especially towards the 'Welfare State', they sometimes wonder whether there is still a place for voluntary action. Excess of officialdom carries its own hazards, notably in the suppression of the individual and his independence. One effect of public welfare that is wholly to the good is the increasing reliance on personal service rather than on money or endowments. This is especially true in Britain of hospital boards and committees, local authority work, and social service agencies. It is equally true that we should regard the promotion of self-help as part of public policy. This indeed is one of the functions of the great Foundations. And further, social investigations and surveys ought to remain among the prime interests of voluntary activity, even when the actual work is undertaken by workers of professional standing. Under this heading one thinks of reports on hospitals, nursing, etc., and in England, the 'Political and Economic Planning' Reports on many diverse subjects.

Up to this point, the United Kingdom voluntary activities and the Government stand in rather an uneasy equilibrium. Looking back over half a century we find that the doctrine of non-interference is still in the saddle, and one occasionally hears the view that any assistance by Government above mere survival 'saps the sturdy independence of the people'. This is a mere gloss today, especially after war and recessions; but at the height of laissez-faire one had to look in vain for either sturdiness or independence. Instead, in England, one had a fever-haunted, slothful race of obligatory parasites. At the other extreme is the sovereign state, fantastically called 'communism'. It is strongly reminiscent of the state described in the Antigone:*

> CREON: Since when do I take my orders from the people of Thebes?
> Haemon: Isn't that rather a childish thing to say?
> CREON: No, I am ruler; responsible only to myself.
> Haemon: A one-man state? What sort of state is that?
> CREON: Why, does not every state belong to its ruler?
> Haemon: Father, you'd be an excellent king . . . upon a desert island.

The difference is that in a democracy men and women become citizens, not by having rights, but by *using* them. Rights

* Sophocles, Antigone.

are not rewards, decorations, or ends in themselves. They are opportunities, instruments through which, freed from repression and tyranny, the citizen may begin to learn his duty. 'The harpist is not made, except by playing the harp, nor the just man save by doing just deeds'.* Citizenship is one of the larger arts; and to teach men and women to do their duties to the State, the only effective plan is to give them duties to do. The foundation of this is voluntary effort. As Beveridge well said:

'The State should encourage voluntary action of all kinds for social advance. . . . It should, in every field of its growing activity, use, where it can, without destroying their freedom and their spirit, the voluntary agencies born of social conscience and of philanthropy. This is one of the marks of a free society.'†

When we come to public health, in essence the voluntary services are a specialised expression of two universal characteristics: the impulse to reach out wherever help is needed, and a disposition to join forces for carrying out a common purpose. Strictly, if we exclude for the moment hospitals and professional organisations which are *ex-officio* health agencies or dedicated to medical care, we can narrow down the definition to this:

An organisation which is administered by an autonomous board or committee which holds meetings, collects funds for its support chiefly from private sources, and spends money, with or without paid workers, in conducting a programme directed primarily to furthering the public health; by providing health services, or education, or by advancing research or legislation to these ends.

The special characteristics of voluntary health activity are these:

(*a*) They are always on the spreading edge of a movement; leaving to statutory authorities what is fully established.

(*b*) They should have enough faith to take risks, and acquiesce if necessary in being a brilliant failure.

(*c*) They should aim at self-extinction when their objective has been reached (e.g., the ten hours' day, women's suffrage, or abolition of the death penalty).

1. The general types of organisation include specific diseases, especially of the social kind, such as tuberculosis, cancer,

* Aristotle, Ethics.
† Beveridge, Lord: 'Voluntary Action'.

diabetes, and venereal disease. Each one of these is a campaign in itself, and is fought with special weapons.

2. Disabilities of special organs or functions, e.g., the blind, the deaf, the cardiac case, crippling disorder, spastics, and poliomyelitis.

3. Conditions affecting the welfare of special groups, or of society itself, e.g., Maternity and Child Health, Family Planning, Mental Hygiene, Alcoholism, Deprived Children, or Problem Families.

4. In order to bring social legislation up-to-date (e.g., marriage and divorce, suicide, homosexuality).

One of the doubts expressed about the National Health Service, when it was introduced, was that it would stifle voluntary effort. This has proved to be completely false as a prediction. In fact, our calculations show that the proportion of voluntary help has increased by over thirty per cent since the Act came into force. The Service provides, in the first place, for the enlistment of voluntary help at the management level. All members of hospital boards, executive councils, and local health authorities are voluntary and unpaid, but they are advised by full-time officials. Voluntary workers are selected for their individual contribution, and need not represent any organisation, whether social or political.

In addition to management, voluntary effort does a great deal to complement the work of the various organs of the health service. Visiting hospitals and their patients is an important part of the functions, and it has been particularly gratifying to see the keen response of voluntary services in the recent development of mental hospitals under new legislation. Numerous local hospital auxiliary associations and other voluntary bodies provide volunteers to visit patients who are otherwise friendless. There are many voluntary associations whose members, sometimes drawing help from local authorities, give assistance to old people and to the handicapped generally. In many cases, as for example spastics and epileptics, the need for official action has not been fully realised until citizens formed societies and associations to act as pioneers, and to shout for help. In fact, legislation for the deaf, the dumb, and the physically handicapped has already made great strides as a direct result of the efforts of voluntary bodies to bring the needs to the public and the legislators.

The story of the Scottish National Blood Transfusion Association is typical of well-directed voluntary effort. Formed in 1940 as a voluntary association, it has so expanded as to depend only to a small extent on private funds. Its real supporters are more than 140,000 members in Scotland alone (pop. 5 million), who enable it to perform its life-saving work by giving blood donations at regular intervals and without payment. In the last ten years the number of blood donations has risen from 40,000 to 118,000 a year.

The principal voluntary organisations are so well-known that it is hardly necessary to describe them in detail. The World Health Organisation has celebrated the first centenary of the Red Cross Society in an admirable booklet which can be obtained from W.H.O.

In addition to the older societies such as the St. John Ambulance Association and the Red Cross, local authorities have had the benefit of co-operation with many voluntary bodies; of these the nursing associations are outstanding. In recent years, especially since the passing of the National Health Service Act, new voluntary associations have entered the field to give assistance in the care of diseases which have recently come predominantly to public notice. Among these are included the care of spastics and the study of conditions that are in some respects obscure, with the object of elucidating these. Voluntary organisations have contributed extensively to research, notably for the study of cancer and certain blood diseases. There has also been a renewed interest in the study of conditions which although not common are yet obscure. Among these may be included conditions which affect mental health, such as mongolism, epilepsy and diseases of the nervous system. The cardiovascular system has recently received special attention, and more recently still advances have been made in the study of the rheumatic diseases.

Speaking more generally, the voluntary organisations have in recent years made distinguished contributions to research and development.

One striking example of the co-operation between voluntary activity and state service of public health care in the Netherlands is that the services are actually carried out by voluntary agencies while the central Government restricts its activities to supervision, regulation and adjustment. This principle means in practice that the public themselves are very deeply concerned in everyday health care through their membership of voluntary agencies. The central Government helps these agencies to carry on their work, mainly by subsidies under certain conditions. This relationship between private initiative and the authorities works most successfully when the subsidies are large enough to develop the service while leaving the enterprise of voluntary bodies unhampered.

The responsibility for national public health rests with the Minister of Social Affairs and Public Health, who is assisted by a Director-General with an administrative staff of well over 50 civil servants and a number of advisory boards.

About 75 per cent of the population are now covered by sickness insurance, either compulsory (in which case employers and workers both contribute 2·1 per cent of the salary), or voluntary. All persons in paid employment earning less than ($1,816) per annum are, with their families, compulsorily insured.

In the Netherlands there are 221 general hospitals, 42 specialist institutions and 43 sanatoria. Seven of these are State hospitals and 41 are municipal establishments; the others are private institutions.

Chapter 10

MEDICINE AS A SOCIAL SCIENCE

In the year 1779 Johann Peter Frank published the first volume of his immense work on medical police. Frank was a fine clinician, but his interests lay especially in community hygiene, and his faith in the efficacy of legislation is touching: 'At present', he says, 'the authorities give themselves more trouble and spend more money in one week in fruitless attempts to apply remedies than would ever be necessary if effort and money were expended to prevent evils through wise ordinances'. Frank was far ahead of his time, but his influence on social medicine was great and lasting. His teaching fell on fertile soil in the person of Andrew Duncan the elder (1744-1828) who founded the Royal Public Dispensary in Edinburgh. In 1798 Duncan presented a memorial to the Patrons of the University of Edinburgh advocating the establishment of a University Chair of Medical Jurisprudence and Medical Police, and in May 1807 George III granted a commission creating the desired professorship with an endowment of a hundred pounds a year. This progressive step did not escape criticism. We are told that when the offending Ministry were turned out of office the Tory party of the day pounced upon this Edinburgh professorship with expressions of virtuous indignation. Spencer Perceval said he was at a loss to understand what the late government could mean by the appointment; he was ignorant, he confessed, of the duty of that professor and could not comprehend what was meant by the science he professed. Perceval was no doubt more interested in his budget, but he might have taken the trouble to read Duncan's memorial which, after dealing in clear outline with the subject of medical jurisprudence, proceeds to enter an eloquent plea for the cause of preventive medicine:

'Of incomparably greater consequence', he writes, 'and more widely extended influence, is the second division of this subject; it regards not merely the welfare of individuals, but the prosperity and security of nations. It is perhaps the most important branch of general police; for its influence is not confined to those whom accidental circumstances bring within its sphere, but extends over the whole population of the State'.

The memorial defines 'medical police' as 'the application of the principles deduced from different branches of medical knowledge for the promotion, preservation, and restoration of general health', and concludes with a brief outline of the subjects for exposition.

No doubt many influences, personal and altruistic, combined to stimulate Dr. Duncan's enthusiasm. The growth of humanity in British politics, so well described by Sir John Simon, and especially the work of John Howard, were part of his everyday knowledge; as an editor and reviewer he was familiar with the steady progress of public health teaching in Germany, and he was certainly influenced by a report, published in 1790 by a committee of the Royal Society of Medicine in Paris—'Nouveau Plan de Constitution pour la Médecine en France'. This committee recommended as one of five principal subjects of the medical curriculum 'the choice of the means most conducive to the preservation of the body in a state of health', and contemplated the appointment of a professor of hygiene. It was pointed out that

> instruction in hygiene and in clinical medicine will be perfectly new institutions in France; for hygiene in the manner in which it has hitherto been taught in the colleges comprehends only a few trivial facts.*

John Gordon Smith, writing in 1824, gives a wider definition:

> The application of medical knowledge to the benefit of man in his social state.

This surely is just what the term means today: the application of Medicine to man in his environment—that is, against the background of his home, his family, his food, and his work and play. A century ago it was distinguished from 'poor law' salvage medicine, the principles of which were as follows:

1. To wait until destitution or sickness is firmly established and then to offer relief.

2. To give as little relief as possible, as late as possible, and for as short a time as possible.

---

* *Medical Commentaries*, Vol. 8 (Edited by Andrew Duncan, Sen.).

3. To tide over the period of affliction by some means which will do nothing to prevent its recurrence.

4. To assume that all distress is temporary, and therefore to rely on purely temporary remedies.

5. To provide services without ensuring that they are distributed to the best advantage of the people as a whole.

In the prospectus of the Edinburgh Public Dispensary, Duncan refers to the General Dispensary in Aldersgate, London, which Lettsom had formed in 1770, and he seems to have derived the idea from there. He makes no mention of George Armstrong's Children's Dispensary, which was established in 1769 in Red Lion Square, London. The Edinburgh Dispensary continued without much change until 1815; it undertook no domiciliary work, and held clinics only two days a week.

Meanwhile other dispensaries were established in Scotland—Kelso, Haddington, Duns, Dundee and Aberdeen. The Kelso scheme was synchronous with that of Duncan in Edinburgh, but the proposal makes no mention of either Duncan or Lettsom. In all probability it derived from Armstrong's Children's Dispensary, for George Armstrong and his brother John, the poet-physician, Andrew Wilson, Sir John Pringle and William Buchan of domestic medicine fame—who were all closely associated with Armstrong's Children's Dispensary—were Roxburghshire men. This venture provided a fair solution to the problem of a rural medical service for an area radiating seven miles from Kelso, domiciliary services and all.

The Aberdeen Dispensary became associated with teaching, and in 1860, in the University prospectus, it was still regarded as an important item in clinical instruction. In Sir John Sinclair's 'Statistical Account of Scotland' (1797) 'several gentlemen of the city' report of it in the following terms:

> The Aberdeen Dispensary was instituted in 1781 for the purpose of attending, at their own homes, such patients as could not be admitted to the Infirmary. It is supported by the bounty of the public, and is under the management of contributors. Dr. Gordon, the present physician, has had charge of it for ten years.
>
> The utility of the institution to the poor will appear from the following abstracts ... But it is calculated to be extremely useful in other respects: namely, as being an excellent school for the education of medical students, and on account of the ample

field it presents for observation and the acquisition of practical knowledge, affording, of course, the best of opportunities for improving the science of medicine. . .

At present, it shall only be observed, that the general principle which pervades and guides the whole of (Dr. Gordon's) practice is to imitate and follow the footsteps of nature, to make art subservient to nature and theory to practice. This method is not new, though of late too much neglected; for the same principle has been the guide of all the great *practical physicians*, both of ancient and modern times. And it is by this method only that the art of physic can be improved and brought to perfection. It is not to be improved by hypotheses and ingenious theories formed in the closet, but by observations accurately made in the chambers of the sick.

William Stokes (Senior) of Dublin, in addition to his great talent as a clinician, was one of the protagonists of public health. As a member of the Royal Sanitary Commission of 1869 he helped to promote the best endeavours in preventive medicine, and in his position on the General Medical Council he was one of the foremost advocates of the creation of a special diploma in public health (Dublin, 1871). His professional life in Dublin was distinguished by his deep interest in the care of the poor and his unselfish devotion to the ideal of state medicine.

Sir Henry Wentworth Acland,* Regius Professor of Medicine in Oxford from 1858 to 1874, represented his University on the General Medical Council for many years and was for a time its president. Like Stokes he was a member of the Royal Sanitary Commission of 1869 and was untiring in his advocacy of social medicine in both teaching and practice. His own words tell of his approach to social medicine as long ago as 1889:

Now we see that the complicated condition of human society with its pressing needs demands such extended estimate of the Physician's functions as to include not only the treatment but the prevention of disease in individuals, in families and in communities, and the difficult problems of comparative National Health. Fifty years ago some older practical men would ridicule a young Physician who gave attention to the health condition of dwellings, or even to hospital construction. In this country the thoughtful medical man working among the poor is now brought into contact with questions foreign to the actual practice of his art, such as out-door relief, medical relief, the employment of

* Acland, Sir Henry 'Letter to a Colleague' 1889.

district nurses, and their relations to the distribution of medical comforts. All these are part of the daily life of some medical men, and those who do not share them ought all the more to have acquired just views concerning them, so as to help on sound public opinion and to create just professional sentiment.

Acland then goes on to urge that students should be given opportunities of studying social conditions at first hand.

Another prominent member of the same Royal Sanitary Commission was Sir Thomas Watson (1792-1882), a leading London physician and Professor of Medicine, also well versed in the ideals of prevention. What was the happy coincidence that brought these three men of forward view into the same counsels, the same vigorous support of the social factor in medicine? The answer is William Pulteney Alison, physician and teacher, of Edinburgh. But let me stand aside and hear others speak:

'William Stokes', writes his son, 'then proceeded to Edinburgh to complete his studies ... There it was that, stimulated by the magnetic influence of Professor Alison, he developed that study of clinical medicine (that) placed him among the pioneers of medical science'. An account of his first interview with Alison is given by Sir Henry Acland in his biographical sketch of Stokes.

> He was walking one wet night down the old Cowgate; he observed a crowd at the entrance to a dark passage: he stopped to see what it could mean; he entered a low room filled with sick poor, Professor Alison being seated among them: he watched the scene: a young man evidently suffering from an advanced fever stepped forward. Alison said: 'Go to your bed, and when I have done here, I will come to you.' (Stokes steps forward and offers to take the man home and to report to Alison how he goes on).

This incident would be in New Town Dispensary about 1824. Later in life William Stokes observed:

> Alison was the best man I ever knew ... It was my good fortune to be very closely connected with him during my student days in Edinburgh and to attend him by day and more often into the night in his visits to the sick poor.

When Acland went to Edinburgh in 1844 he at once began attending lectures and accompanying Dr. Alison round the wards of the infirmary. In 1846 Alison agreed to take Acland into his house as a resident pupil. The biographer says 'the debt which he owed morally and intellectually to Alison was seldom absent from his speech'. He gave the name Alison to his eldest son.

Sir Thomas Watson paid high compliment to Alison through the excellent manuscript notes of his lectures, taken in 1821 and still extant—the only MS notes of Watson's that seem to have been cherished by him!

About the time of the Report (T.C. 1840) some useful publications on the sanitary conditions of Glasgow and Edinburgh appeared . . . in relation to the latter, a treatise by that zealous philanthropist and able physician, Dr. W. P. Alison, and all who have the pleasure of knowing him can speak of his sterling worth and earnest ability, and his unwearied exertions on behalf of the poor of the city of Edinburgh.[1]

W. P. Alison entered Edinburgh College in 1803 and studied both arts and medicine. He was a keen pupil of Dugald Stewart, and his attainments in philosophy were so high that at one time Stewart is said to have hoped that Alison would succeed him in the Chair. In 1811, however, he graduated M.D. and soon began to settle down to his chosen profession. The New Town Dispensary was formed in 1815 and Alison was at once associated with its work as a physician. The new dispensary was soon at loggerheads with the old, and it is clear that it was formed as a protest against the inadequate service rendered by the latter. This dispensary introduced domiciliary services—maternity, daily clinics, and a resident staff for emergency calls. The area was divided into districts, each with a physician, and the students were given district responsibilities. A good working association was formed with the various charitable organisations—the Society for the Relief of the Destitute Sick, the Society for Clothing the Industrious Poor, and the like. Needless to add, the New Town Dispensary was copying from its older rival the system of using the service as a means of teaching. Alison also used it for the collection of social statistics and for epidemiological investigations.

The quarterly medical reports of the dispensary (published in the Edinburgh Medical Journal, 1817-1819) were in great part written by Alison; they contained important contributions to knowledge of fevers, and still supply basic material for the history of epidemics. They also contain observations on small-pox modified by vaccination, which was then little known. In 1820 Alison was appointed to the Chair of Medical Jurisprudence and Medical Police and held that office for two years.

Again, in his brilliant report on the causation of fevers Alison puts his finger unerringly on the conditions within the home—such as overcrowding and dirt—and makes light of the noxious influences of irrigated meadows and dunghills:

> (I propose to) state the grounds of my belief, first, that the contagious fever of Edinburgh does not originate in a malaria generated in the manner above stated; and secondly, that there is a much better prospect of preventing the introduction, and checking the diffusion of a disease to which a large proportion of the lower orders in Edinburgh are particularly liable, by other means of improving their conditions, and particularly by a more liberal and better managed provision against the destitution of the unemployed, or partially or wholly disabled poor, than by any measure directed merely to the removal of these nuisances.

It was in personal qualities that Alison was outstanding. That he acquired a very large consulting practice goes without saying, but it is more noteworthy that he carried out his hospital work with a profound sense of the value of the patient as a person. He was unremitting in his care of poor folk, both in the Infirmary and in visits to their homes, in spite of ever-increasing public duties.

Alison's greatest contribution to the welfare of his fellow men was the outcome of his zeal for social betterment. His pamphlet 'Observations on the Management of the Poor in Scotland, and Its Effects on the Health of the Great Towns' (Edinburgh, 1840) is only one expression of his pervading influence on his own generation and more especially on those young men whom he sent out as teachers and practitioners of social medicine. This is not a vague or idle statement; it can be shown that one cohort of students after another left the University with an undying sense of the practical importance of Alison's teaching and a determination to apply it to their own life-work. The book entitled 'The Physician as Naturalist' (1889) contains 'Addresses and Memoirs bearing on the history and progress of medicine chiefly during the last 100 years'. It is by Sir William Tennent Gairdner. A whole chapter is headed 'Dr. Alison'. It is 'a tribute to the memory of a valued teacher, true friend, a great and good man' so esteemed by 'very many pupils of his in all parts of the world'.

There is a remarkable passage in an address, dated 1866, by Dr. Halliday Douglas—on the character of Alison he says:

> The well known observations on the pathology of scrofulous diseases and on the origin of tubercle, first read to the Medico-Chirurgical Society in 1822, are pre-eminently distinguished by the philanthropic character of Alison's practical writings, and of his bent towards public or *social medicine*. In themselves the observations have an intrinsic value on account of the very complete exposition he gives of the predisposing circumstances and exciting causes of tuberculous disease.

James Burn Russell was born in Glasgow in 1837. After a distinguished career as a student he graduated M.D. at Glasgow University in 1862. He was the first medical superintendent of the Parliamentary Road Fever Hospital in Glasgow, and continued in that office until his appointment as Medical Officer of Health for the City in 1872, in succession to Gairdner. In 1898 he accepted office as medical member of the Local Government Board for Scotland, and served in that capacity until his death in 1904. Russell was a member of Gairdner's first class, and it is not difficult to trace the influence of a teacher who had himself served under Professor Alison. In an account of hospital provision for infectious disease Russell makes this comment:

> These dismal facts in the experience of Glasgow and other large Scotch towns were not passing unobserved by men capable of extracting a healing medicine from their bitter fruit. Drs. Cowan and Perry in Glasgow, and Alison in Edinburgh, were such, and their names will always deserve honourable mention in the records of a philanthropic and philosophic public policy. Three suggestions of measures of primary importance for the public health and general social well-being were derived from the condition of affairs which I have described, and which were urged with the greatest ability and perseverance, by every channel which could reach the intelligence of the public and the legislature, until they ultimately passed into definite enactments. As Dr. Alison pointed out, 'The Statute Law of Scotland *requires* the heritors, ministers and elders of parishes, and the magistrates of burghs, to make provision for the needful sustentation of all aged poor and impotent persons, to enable them to live unbeggared,

and to tax and stint the inhabitants, when necessary, for this purpose'.*

There was a good deal in common between Alison and Russell. Both were men of high integrity with a devouring passion for social medicine. Both derived their knowledge from exhaustive personal effort in visiting slums, and both were moved to indignation and action by what they saw. Alison, I think, was the greater doctor and possessed the more striking personality. Russell could put more venom into his pen, but was not very effective in speech, except in the swift passages of conversation. He is the child of his time in sentimental expression, but far above his age in bitter irony. In his description of the children of the City, for example, he deploys all his forces:

In this aspect of play consider the position of our city children. They are impelled by a restless, ceaseless instinct, and not by the Devil, as the landlords and the police seem to think. Pent up in common stairs and in back courts, without a bit of space which they can call their own, their play inevitably becomes in great part mischief. What can a poor boy do but pull bricks out of the walls of the ashpit to build houses with, or climb upon its roof and tear the slates off to make traps for the city sparrows? If they fly kites, the policeman cuts the string: if they dig holes in the courts to play at marbles, the factor denounces them to the police: if they play ball against the wall, the policeman grabs the ball: if they make slides on the pavement, he puts salt on them: if they try to swim in the river, they are almost poisoned by the sewage, and when they come out, it is to find the man in blue waiting for them beside their clothes: if they pitch a wicket on an empty building site, the birl of the well known whistle stops the game before they have completed their innings. The girls are no better off. As you feel your way along the dark lobbies, blinded by the light you have just left behind you, you stumble over them playing at houses. As you ascend the stairs you have to pick your way through their assortment of broken dishes and odds and ends with which they are reproducing their meagre experiences of housekeeping and shopping.†

This is not the time of day when one can afford to present the character of a hero, to estimate his influence on his time and generation and then call it a day. I believe that Alison deserves

* Russell, J. B. (Memorial Volume), p. 79.
† Russell, J. B., The Children of the City, Edinburgh Health Society, 1886.

eternal recognition as the pioneer in social medicine, and that Scotland ought not to neglect the work of its great men.

In the twentieth century the first important light was shed by an American physician, Dr. Richard C. Cabot of Boston, who introduced medical social workers into the teaching of students. This was in fact a much greater advance than could have been anticipated, as it opened the doors to practical studies by the students in their public health course, not only of health needs but also of social conditions under which the population lived.

This work was carried forward to a remarkable extent by Professor René Sand of Belgium who, in addition to his teaching, wrote a basic study under the title 'The Advance to Social Medicine'. Rene Sand was himself a brilliant teacher, and in addition to his social interests his name will always be remembered as one of the pioneers of world health. He was Chairman of the Technical Preparatory Committee in 1946 which led to the setting up of the World Health Organisation.

In England a great advance was made through the agency of the Nuffield Foundation. The appointment of a brilliant clinician, Professor John A. Ryle, to the first Nuffield Chair of Social Medicine—in Oxford—was a notable achievement which had repercussions throughout the country, both in teaching and in practice. Ryle's contributions to the development of social medicine were in themselves very great, but even more important was his influence on the study of social factors in medicine and the promotion of ideas which led to the establishment of other University Chairs.

REFERENCE

[1]Ikin, T. Ingham (1851): On the Progress of Public Hygiene, *Proc. med. surg. J.*, p. 569.

Chapter 11

HEALTH EDUCATION

One telling advantage of health education is that its methods can be adapted to the needs of communities at their very early stages of development. There is no overall course which must be taught, and so each country, each authority, on taking up the subject, is free to organise a scheme of teaching to fit its own background, and the traditions and culture of its people. It is essential that trained and experienced staff should experiment in each area with different methods of teaching and presentation, in order to find out what level of instruction and what types of background illustration are most suitable for those who are learning. There are a number of rules of the game which have been found out through the process of trial and error.

In the first place it is important for the authorities to realise that health education is an essential part of modern teaching whether at school or before an adult audience. The second feature is that in one sense the subject of health education is a new one and offers wide scope for experimentation. Teaching people about health is as old as the hills but a well defined course in health education, appropriate for various nations, especially the so-called emerging nations, is something that demands the careful training of teachers.

In earlier times health education had gone through two distinct phases. In the eighteenth century there arose a great interest in health under the leadership of France and French philosophy. It was closely associated with what has been called the growth of humanistic ideals. The movement became international in Europe. On its dark side it was accompanied by revolution in which France also took a leading part. In spite of this, the advantages had far reaching effects, because new ideals were put forward. This was noteworthy in Britain through the writings of Locke on the one side and religious revivals on the other—not because either of these attempted to deal specifically with education and health, but because they reached towards a much larger population than ever before. The work of John and Charles Wesley, in particular, extended humane ideals to the poor, and its educational value was incomparable. Medicine also played its part, especially towards the end of the century when the new philosophy inspired greater care for the poor, including the establishment of foundling homes, hospitals and dispensaries for children. These have been previously noted in these pages but attention must be drawn at this point most carefully to the educative value of social progress, notably to the work of men like John Howard.

Unfortunately the early movements towards humanism had to remain in abeyance for many years because of the tendency throughout Europe towards revolutionary wars, and the industrial revolution, as it was called, began to do its worst shortly after the end of the Napoleonic Wars. It was not until the middle of the nineteenth century that the humanitarian spirit began to revive and raise its head above the din of laissez-faire economics.

At this period the causes of the new development were quite different and indeed spread much more generally through the people. The rise in the position of women, particularly their appointment on Boards of Guardians, their interest in social studies, and their increasing association with public affairs, such as health services and the care of infants and young children, gave a fresh stimulus to the study of social conditions and in many cases a more liberal outlook. Many women of intellect arose to the new challenge, and the world owes a great debt to the pioneers of education, medicine and social work on both sides of the Atlantic.

In addition to this forward movement there were improvements in the attitude towards the less privileged, and a growing unwillingness to contemplate the perpetuation of gross anomalies between one class and another. The rise of the Fabian movement is a case in point because it contributed in large measure to legislation for the benefit of workers in their homes, mothers and children, and the aged and afflicted. Indeed, this was the main reason why the twentieth century opened with a new concept of community health, and a keen desire to promote it by voluntary effort, passing ultimately to legislation. The growth of mental health work as a voluntary movement is a splendid illustration of this, and examples could be multiplied, in the progress of school health, in maternal and infant care, and in a fresh consideration of the needs of the elderly.

The twentieth century began with a new spirit largely because men and women of independent minds were studying social problems objectively and scientifically. They were soon impressed by the enormous wastage of child life, much of which arose from personal rather than from environmental defects which had been so much before the eyes of the previous century. Movements on behalf of child protection gained steadily in strength during the first decade and won statutory recognition in a remarkable series of Acts dealing with midwives, the care of school children, the protection of children from injury or neglect, and infant welfare. This phase has now passed and there has been a rich harvest, but today we are in serious danger of falling into the same morass as the legislators of a century ago, because the movement for personal health is now lacking a single great directive aim. It is not growing as an organism, but only in response to specific pressures here and there and not as a result of any large and inspiring social policy. This criticism may be countered by the snail's pace argument of 'one thing at a time'. . . 'not too fast'. . . 'slow and sure'. Indeed this argument is sound up to a point, provided that there is a plan ready to cover the whole, but it is unsound in so far as it means 'little by little', without any plan.

One of the sources of difficulty at the present time, especially in some of the countries in the course of development, is that two health issues which were really separate are in danger of becoming confused. The advancement of personal health as a branch of preventive medicine has been made effective during the past forty years in the industrialised countries, and there has been a large volume of legislation to support what is broadly known as 'public health'. The statutes dealing with midwifery, maternity, child welfare and epidemic disease, and the great bulk relating to the poor law, are part and parcel of preventive medicine and reflect faithfully the attitude of the public mind towards the health of the individual. In addition, the immense mass of social legislation dealing with pensions, industrial insurance and general insurance against sickness are all consciously directed to the promotion of health by preventing diseases and destitution.

In the field of mental health recent legislation breaks away from the concept of mental disorder as a condition requiring compulsory segregation in the interests of the community; it begins to recognize mental disorder as an illness just like other illnesses, susceptible of treatment for the benefit of the individual patient. More recently some countries seem to be changing their attitude towards drug addiction and are no longer regarding it as a crime to be dealt with by means of restraint or other penal laws. All these, and many other advances in preventive medicine, are worthy contributions to health; and our national and local authorities are playing a notable part in implementing these provisions.

All the progressive measures to which I refer relate to preventive medicine and take only an indirect interest in the promotion of health. This is the second issue, more fundamental than the first but less clearly perceived than either treatment or prevention. Nevertheless it is the logical outcome of a social policy which begins with treatment and proceeds to prevention. This sequence of events can readily be seen in the recent history of some of the emerging nations, especially in Africa.

The first need was medical care and the demand was for the construction of hospitals. In the same way we can see this sequence of events among the older communities in the evolution of the school medical service. In the first stage it was discovered that the physical fitness of the nation was not what it ought to be. Attention was then very properly turned to the condition of growing children and this procedure disclosed an appalling amount of sickness in the course of school medical inspection. The immediate result of inspection was to reveal that a large amount of sickness, and in consequence loss of school attendance, was due to minor conditions which respond readily to treatment. The progressive clearing up of uncleanliness, skin diseases, and other mild infections improved matters considerably, but at the same time uncovered the hidden fact that the stream of unhealthy children entering school for the first time was in no way diminished. It was clearly necessary to go further back into child life and to attack disease nearer its source. This splendid contribution to the community showed clearly that the urgent need was for education in health, and the nursery school in particular, as a place where actual living goes on, has shown how health education can become as much part of everyday life as eating and sleeping.

Planned education for health falls into three divisions, all of which are important functions of the health authorities:

1. Education of the expectant mother and of the mother with a young infant. This is carried out through ante-natal care and the infant welfare centre.

2. Education of the child through infancy, early life, and school age, in personal health and social co-operation.

3. Education of adolescent boys and girls in personal and social hygiene, including the responsibilities of parenthood.

This extensive programme is not nearly so difficult as it looks, because it makes use of existing materials, that is, of facilities that health authorities possess or which are immediately available through such bodies as the Central Council for Health Education. In fact it is true to say that one of the reasons for diffidence in bringing forward a programme of this kind is that it is so simple, obvious and logical. It is hard to persuade people today that we are not already carrying out health education. Nevertheless, education for health is in most areas a neglected field, and many national and local authorities do not realise even today that it is the most economical and effective agent of preventive medicine.

In a number of countries the public health services are closely allied, both centrally and locally, to the educational system. In many ways this is a wise arrangement because the two services have much in common. Both are primarily concerned with teaching and require the use of techniques appropriate for group work. The essence of the educational method consists in maintaining a just balance between individual teaching and class instruction, and its success depends upon understanding and confidence between home and school. The schools do indeed offer instruction, but it is the happy co-operation with the parents that give it life and purpose. Similar principles are applicable to the practice of public health. It is in its essence an educational service, and it employs both individual and group teaching adapted as need be to its special purposes. Its aim is to promote better and healthier ways of living.

The means it uses are: first to protect the environment, and secondly to teach the people patiently, simply and often. The success of public health teaching as a service to the community depends upon its gaining the confidence of the people so that they learn almost unaware. Health measures are most effective when they are readily absorbed into the everyday routines of living, and the health officer is most successful when he creates silent social revolutions. As Lowndes* pointed out:

Much modern politico-social writing is accordingly vitiated by the tendency to demand social revolution without first pausing to discover how far and how fast the silent social revolution effected by educational changes has proceeded...

It is vain to expect to educate the people of this country except by gradually inducing them to educate themselves... The people perhaps cannot give guidance, but they can give life, which is even more valuable than guidance. With the people what we may do may be imperfect, without them we shall probably do little or nothing.

*Lowndes, A. M. "The Silent Social Revolution".

Chapter 12

CARE OF THE AGED

The contribution of public health practice to the care of the aged and the understanding of their problems has grown enormously in recent years, and indeed it is hard to find specific references to the subject in the literature of health services except in the past twenty years. This is not to imply that the aged, in sickness and in health, have been previously neglected or ignored. There are countless references throughout the centuries to the blessings and to the hardships of old age. It was Sophocles who said: 'And, last of all, age claims him for her own—age, dispraised, infirm, unsociable, unfriended, with whom all woe abides.' There were others who saw the brighter side: Socrates, for example, rejoiced in conversation with the aged:

> To tell you the truth, Cephalus, I am very fond of conversation with elderly folk. They have gone before us on the road over which perhaps we also shall have to travel, and I think we ought to try to learn from them what the road is like—whether rough and difficult or smooth and easy. And now that you have arrived at that period of life which poets call 'the threshold of age' there is no one whose opinion I would more gladly ask.[1]

Examples from the past could be multiplied, and the attitudes of the older civilisations to the elders make a fascinating enquiry. A great deal depended upon whether they were regarded as within the family group, and in certain races and periods the elderly wielded an immense amount of power. Indeed, there is no doubt that their strength and happiness was largely dependent upon their usefulness, that is, on the amount of influence which was accorded to them on account of the reputed wisdom of years. Dependent old age, without influence, must have been unhappy at all times. As Doctor Johnson put it: 'There is no state more contrary to the dignity of wisdom than perpetual and unlimited dependence, in which understanding lies useless, and every motion is received from external impulse.'[2]

In a book published in 1930, with the title 'Salvaging Old Age', one of the joint authors noted that she had made a vain search through the literature of health and social science for something definite, something positive, about the period of old age, which she was proceeding to study. Then she turned to the writings of the psychologists, only to find that their views of senescence were sombre, indeed hopeless, and distinctly materialistic. Much of the general literature up to the nineteenth century took a similar view about old age; as Francis Bacon put it in a nutshell: 'Men of age object too much, consult too long, adventure too little, relent too soon, and seldom drive business home to the full period, but content themselves with a mediocrity of success.'[3]

All this seems to point to the urgent need for attention to the behaviour problems of the old, and it is clear that the increasing devotion offered during the past generation or so to the medical and social care of the aged and infirm is a great and necessary step forward in the realm of public health practice. It is common knowledge that many old people become just as troublesome as difficult children, but until recently we have been shy of facing the issue. The reasons for diffidence are evident: the dignity of age, the long tradition of reverence sanctioned by creed and custom, the authority to which the elders cling, no doubt far too long in many cases; and above all, the reputed wisdom of experience. All these not only prevent us from taking health measures, but even tend to preclude us from studying and analysing the less desirable features of senility. In ordinary conversation it is embarrassing even to talk about the egoism, the fierce clinging to power, the petulance, the readiness to take offence, and the utter childishness that sometimes mar the grave countenance of age. We have around us a number of noble ruins which merit preservation, but nevertheless require to be trimmed and kept within bounds.

What might be called 'the cult of old age' developed in strength during the nineteenth century, more as a sentiment than as a practical belief. 'Old age hath yet his honour and his toil',[4] Tennyson says; and Browning, going further in his enthusiasm, urged that 'the best is yet to come'.[5] Hardy was ready to observe that:

> Sophocles, Plato, Socrates,
>   Gentlemen,
> Pythagoras, Thucydides,
> Herodotus and Homer—yea,
> Clement, Augustin, Origen,
> Burnt brightlier towards their setting day,
>   Gentlemen. [6]

and this was no doubt a great source of comfort to the old man whose temperament could not usually be described as jolly.

It is true that in more ways than one the first decade of the present century deserves to be called 'the age of the child'. The great era of environmental sanitation, which reached its summit in 1875, was now giving way to a better concept of the prevention of sickness both in individuals and in the community. This movement led to a number of important regulations for the care of children and for their protection against the hazards of life. The child had come into the world of public care, and practical public health by now included the prevention of disease in childhood and the realities of health promotion. In England, for example, legislation for the prevention of cruelty to children reached the Statute Book as early as 1908, and in the United States the foundations of child guidance were laid at about the same period and the movement widely extended in the years following the first world war. It may well be that care of the aged, as a public concern, grew out of the preventive care and guidance of children. In the introduction to the book already referred to, 'Salvaging Old Age', one of the authors says:

> This work, which has so often been spoken of as original, really evolved out of work previously done in a similar field. When, in 1920, Dr. Martin established a child guidance clinic for preschool-age children—the first of its kind in this part of the world—it was undertaken as a piece of preventive mental hygiene. . . Those of us who were to have the privilege of working in child guidance had been trained for the purpose and it needed no very astute observer to note that we were extremely well pleased with ourselves to be engaged in this then pioneer work. An agreement had been made that after each group of twenty children had been worked with, we were to meet with Dr. Martin for discussion as to cause of complaint, classification of data, and progress achieved. Eager to report on our findings we held the first conference after having attended to but ten children, and came

face to face with our first surprise. Cases Nos. 1, 3 and 9 suffered from temper spells, marked preferential activity in all fields, and tyranny, respectively, each in imitation of a grandparent living in the home of the child. On the card of the tyrannical child, after the word CAUSE, the home investigator had written the initials O.I., which stood for Old Ironsides—an alias she had given to the resistant grandparent whose behaviour had been the child's model. We were given one week, until the next conference, to come to a conclusion as to what was to be done in such cases. In spite of much thought and discussion and speculation on our part the verdict was unanimous—Old Ironsides must be scrapped, our ideas being of the herd variety. Our second surprise came when Dr. Martin reversed the decision with: 'not scrapped but salvaged'.[7]

In this way they set out on a voyage of discovery, but for the next six years the new job of restoring the old claimed only the time that could be snatched from child guidance. The workers themselves had first to learn to adapt their outlook to the needs of the elderly, and to find out what type of work might be appropriate for them. One of the workers put in many months as a hand in a local factory, while another devoted her energies to serving in a large department store. The third took as her study the old folk who spend their time sitting around in the parks, and the fourth chose the social agencies which specialised in the relief of the aged. Added to the list were personal friends and acquaintances of the workers who thus became valuable guinea-pigs in the experiment. Altogether some 263 cases were dealt with—between the ages of sixty and eighty-six at the time of entry. The clinics held by Dr. Martin were free, and were organised in the evenings for those still at work. Men and women were seen separately, in order to encourage freedom of speech:

> When with the men, the women assumed an artificial attitude and were often constrained in their expression, while the men either preened themselves or became somewhat timid.

Dr. Martin tells the story of how she chose the subject 'Salvaging Old Age' for a series of lectures which she had been invited to give in San Francisco. Angry remonstrations came from the sponsors on the ground that the title would not attract audiences, but she stuck to her guns. At the first lecture, attended by about twenty men and women, there was an hour's discussion on problems of rehabilitation; and when the time

L

came for the closing lecture of the series, the audience of two hundred clearly showed that the old resistance had gone, and that the next step in adult education—the study of the care of the aged—would take far less time to filter through the community than had been anticipated. And so the event has proved, in many countries of the world.

In those days, thirty years ago, there were certainly stirrings of a new interest in the care of the aged; but it was more than interest alone; there were signs of rethinking the problems in terms of health rather than sickness, and of suitable employment in addition to static care. I recollect that in England in the year 1930 a number of health officers and their colleagues in the welfare services had begun to examine the old poor law institutions, at the time when they were transferred from the 'Guardians of the Poor' to the local county and county borough councils under the provisions of the Local Government Act of 1929. This Act transferred responsibility for the care of the poor from the old 'Guardians' to the public health authorities. My colleague, W. H. Abbott, the Public Assistance Officer, and I set ourselves the task of reporting upon the old poor law hospitals; and here is a brief excerpt from our report on this subject, dated June 1930:

> We have examined with great care the present type of accommodation provided for the aged and infirm, and we have come to the conclusion that it is not satisfactory either in extent or in quality. At the present time the aged and infirm are accommodated either in the House along with other classes of case, or in the Infirmary—in the institutions where a separate block has been provided. There are grave objections to both types. With regard to the House the wards are in the majority of instances very unsuitable for the aged: they are frequently difficult of access—sometimes one, sometimes two, floors above ground level and reached only by narrow stairs. There is insufficient provision against fire, and in not a few cases the staff find it convenient to keep these patients in bed, or at least confined to the ward, simply on account of the difficulty of moving them up and down stairs, when from the health point of view fresh air, sunshine, and a little exercise would add greatly to the happiness and well-being of the patients.
>
> In the second place the Infirmary, however modern in construction, is not a suitable place for patients who are inmates

of the institutions merely on account of age and infirmity, without the presence of definite and disabling physical disease. Aged persons who are kept in an infirmary are apt to be looked upon, and to look upon themselves, as hospital cases, even though they require no medical or nursing attention. They are considered as persons laid aside finally until their release by death. This, it appears to us, is not the right point of view. These aged persons, even when old age is accompanied by some degree of infirmity such as impaired sight and hearing, rheumatism, deformity and the like, should nevertheless be encouraged to consider themselves alive enough to enjoy the opportunity of sitting and talking together during the day, around a fire in winter time, and in summer on a pleasant verandah facing a garden where flowers and trees will give delight. We feel, therefore, that the type of provision which should be aimed at when any new structural work can be undertaken, is not an Infirmary block, nor a Hospital, but a building on the bungalow principle, equipped with a pleasant day-room and a series of small wards (say, six beds at most in each) with a wide verandah running along its length and facing South.[8]

A short time ago Dr. George Silver brought to our attention a book published in 1881 with the title 'Fifty Years and Beyond'. This book was written chiefly for evangelical purposes, and carries the sub-title 'Gathered Gems for the Aged'. 'This volume', says the preface, 'has been prepared for persons of mature and advanced years. . . . There are numerous volumes for children and youth. Books abound for young men and young women in life's various relations and pursuits, but only a few volumes have ever been prepared for those who are passing through the afternoon and the evening of life. . . . The author has sought to enrich its pages by such articles as will impart instruction and comfort to the aged, teaching how the later years of life may be spent, so that they shall constitute the happiest and most useful of all life's periods.'[9]

The first chapter of the book deals with the hygiene of old age. Its author presents a gloomy picture of the growing disabilities of poor men after the age of sixty, with the assurance that the downward trend often begins at a much earlier age. He quotes the saying of Benjamin Rush that he had never met a person over eighty whose ancestors were not long-lived.

The next article, written for another purpose by Joseph R.

Richardson, M.D., Professor of Hygiene in the University of Pennsylvania, takes a similar view:

> For the purpose of aiding my elderly readers who are not yet tired of life, and who desire to *grow old* comfortably for some years more, perhaps even to see what the year 1900 A.D. will do for science, art, and humanity, I will briefly glance at the symptoms of bodily decay, in the order in which they are apt to make their onset, and in the same concise way point out how to diminish their interference with the power of life, and their disturbances of health.

The selection of signs and symptoms is sensible: decay of the teeth and the need for skilled dental care 'to prolong for many years the usefulness of decayed teeth, and finally to substitute for them artificial molars and incisors, which perform their vicarious office with wonderful success.'

Another important change, Richardson says, liable to accompany advancing years, is the excessive deposit of fat; and he goes on to point out that this tendency may be diminished by attention to diet. Finally, almost as an afterthought, the author closes his remarks on the subject by mentioning that 'calcareous or chalky degeneration of the arteries, etc., is a common and serious mode of decay in advanced life, due in part, perhaps, to errors in diet'.

Much more stress is laid on the failure of muscular power, in which it is indicated that this takes place in the involuntary muscles and, 'occurring consequently in the heart and the semi-voluntary muscles which inflate the lungs by expanding the chest, renders the vital functions of the respiration and of the circulation of the blood feeble and imperfectly performed'. Rather significantly he adds that, of course, we have no means of examining the heart and seeing whether in any particular individual this waste has begun. The real conclusion is that people can never enjoy good health while they suffer from constipation, a vice much more prevalent than is generally believed.

A closing wave of the hand is offered to deterioration of brain and nerve structure, with the kindly thought that life and intellectual vigour would often be prolonged by judicious changes of occupation and of scene, notably in foreign travel.

Suggestions about the preservation of nerve and mental

health are afforded a special chapter prepared by J. S. Jewell, M.D. Following upon a short description of the structure and modes of action of the nervous system, Dr. Jewell proceeds to indicate that disorder or disease of the nervous system may be produced by over-action or over-excitation, mainly due to loss of the contractile power of the arteries in the brain, leading to endarteritis and consequent enlargement and sluggishness of the vessels. This in turn is associated with aneurysm and cerebral haemorrhage, and even short of such dire results leads to sleeplessness and various other symptoms of congestion caused by permanent dilation of the blood vessels.

The final chapter of this book was written by the Rev. Robert W. Patterson, D.D., Professor of Christian Evidences and Ethics in the Presbyterian Theological Seminary of the North-west. In a very interesting essay the writer expresses his view that the physical decline begins ordinarily some ten years earlier than the mental—and he places the former at 49 years. This is not quite so hard as the famous apothegm of William Osler, but it comes pretty near the bone.

The comments on mental effort in advanced years are certainly more encouraging than those of the physicians.

'Some men', the writer says,

'go out of business, and others abandon their professional pursuits, as soon as advanced age begins to come on, having acquired sufficient means for the support of themselves and their families, or from the sheer desire of rest. Such a policy is most unwise; for the reason that we all need some pressure upon us as a spur to continued mental activity. And without a persistent use of the mental faculties they will inevitably lose their vigour before the time. I have observed for many years that those who relinquish their pursuits while they have yet health and strength for the prosecution of their callings, are accustomed to suffer loss by the rapid decline of both their physical and intellectual powers. A man who has no regular duties to perform will seldom tax himself with efforts which he may easily neglect. He may resolve to keep up his reading and studies, or to give his attention to the exciting questions of the time. But his thinking will grow increasingly languid, and he will gradually sink into the habit of recurring to the past for the food of his mind, and will soon fall behind the active generation in point of intellectual brightness and ready intelligence. I would say to every elderly man: 'Die with the harness on'. It may not be wise to keep the shoulder under the same heavy burdens that were borne in middle life. But it is wise, relaxing somewhat the tension of the mind, to hold on in bearing such responsibilities as will require the highest degree of mental exertion as may be put forth without a sense of oppression to mind or body. And the more agreeable one can make his regular employments the better for his mental health.'

We may now turn to modern times, noting the more cheerful title of 'Five Hundred Over Sixty'.[10] This community survey of ageing was carried out jointly by the Department of Health of New York City, Cornell University's Medical College and Social Science Research Center, and the Russell Sage Foundation. Answers were obtained through personal interviews with a sample of 500 individuals sixty years of age or over residing in the area served by the Kips Bay—Yorkville Health Center, which caters for the needs of some 250,000 people. The Health Centre had developed the general health services and had done a great deal for the children and young adults, but almost nothing for the old people of the district. It is frankly admitted that the reason was simple—'we did not know what to do'. Not knowing what the essential needs of the aged were, the Health Centre wisely created a committee to find out; and this is the origin of this fine and comprehensive report, which is in a true sense a pioneering effort—a prototype rather than a model, as the authors indicate.

From the start of the survey it is clear that there are few precedents. In fact, it is evident that while the problems are, many of them, of long standing, it is only in recent years that they have been tackled systematically. The rapid growth of this group, and the new problems forced upon the community by their presence, has rightly created for them a public health service with a genuine sense of the need for integration. The study covered five hundred persons over the age of sixty who were living in the open—that is, not in institutions. Four specific problems were exposed: personal adjustment; factors relating directly to health; the use of community health services; and attitudes towards health and social centres. It is no part of this essay to report upon or summarise this work, but it is of such significance in the story of the care of aged persons as a measure of practical public health that it occupies a special place in current history. It is significant, even with a selective choice, that out of the large bibliography of 389 titles given in an appendix only a handful dated from before 1950 and but one before 1945. Nevertheless, an examination of the earlier literature of study shows that little interest was in fact attached to the problem until the last decade, and then the floods were let loose. This does not mean that everyone rushed into print because of a passion to be in the fashion, although this cannot be entirely excluded; it rather indicates a sudden awakening to a new social need which had not hitherto been regarded as an aspect of community health, still less the subject for a public health department. Once a barrier is broken down there is a great flood of activity. We ought therefore to look at trends and programmes as set out in this community study. It was found at a very early stage that there were few health or welfare agencies whose programmes were specifically designed to meet the needs of older people. Many services, it is true, were open to all groups; but it is notorious that the aged are often reluctant to use them. We may discuss the reasons for this later, but at the moment the plain fact is that in most areas the existing health and social services, however well designed for the community as a whole, are not in many instances appropriate to satisfy the felt but unexpressed needs of the old. This has been brought out again and again in specially directed enquiries. Two aspects stand out clearly enough: that there is a fundamental shyness among many older people which may be presented as such or concealed in a certain aggressiveness represented in phrases like: 'I have always stood on my own feet, and I don't want charity now'. This is understandable, and it cannot be met merely by saying 'Don't be silly', because it is not silly. On the other hand there is today, as ever, a genuine feeling that youth, or at least the earning period, should be served first, and that age, however deserving, ought to be left to the second place, especially when the purse is limited to serving the prime needs.

The possibility of prolonging effective working capacity of the individual is a subject which requires careful consideration. We have endeavoured to prevent death at the earlier ages, but have devoted little attention to combating the prevalent idea that an individual is too old at fifty for any new employment; yet as a nation we have spent much money on the training of each person, and it would appear to be economically a mistake to get so little out of the individual as we do at present.[11]

These words were written in the year 1911 by the Health Officer of the city of Birmingham, England. If we make a graceful gesture towards substituting the figure of 65 for 50, the same problem is with us today. The burden on the wage earner is even heavier in these days of the high cost of medical care. In recent years, as we have seen, a great mass of literature, medical, economic and social, has arisen about the care of the aged; but in a good deal of the writing it is still assumed that the difficulty can be met by keeping elderly people at their work for a few years longer, and indeed in many forms of employment the retiring age has been raised to 65 or even higher. This proposal is disarmingly simple, even if we suppose that the group so dealt with is passed as physically fit. But it does not really face the issue. It is true that arrangements of this kind, intelligently pursued, may soften the harsh edges of retirement, but it does nothing to meet the problem of those who have in fact retired, whatever the age.

The balance of youth and age is of special importance when skill of eye and ear have to be poised against the very real advantages of wisdom and judgment. Yet it gives a clue to one form of action, and this is based on the observation that the younger excel in speed and skill and the older in counsel. The pressure exercised by the young is partly due to the fact that they have generally increasing home commitments; and the elders might fruitfully take the hint and relax in the presence of decreasing external responsibilities. If this were merely a matter of years, the problem might be solved along these lines. But just as the child has special characteristics and aptitudes which differ from those of the adult, so too have the aged their special skills and interests. We should consider this point positively and scientifically, just as we ought to do with those who are seeking a job for the first time. The essential thing is to find out what jobs an elderly man or woman can do well—perhaps even better than the younger folk. For example, it has been shown that old workers in skilled trades can be relied on to an increasing extent for accuracy, so long as they are not hurried. The pace must be slowed. Again, under good conditions of work the attendance of the elderly at their jobs, and especially their time-keeping, is often exemplary. The cynic might say that this is because they feel insecure, but that is no argument against their employment. The essential point is that we ought to find proper criteria for testing the capacity, both physical and mental, of those who have gone over the retiring line. The elderly man or woman should be given encouragement to go on, but at the same time made clearly to understand that this is not a matter of charity or sentiment, but of capacity. In other words, the arrangements for testing should be similar to those used with success in the case of the crippled. We should regard the old person as a candidate for new employment and, although much can be said against an arbitrary retiring age, it has the undoubted advantage of being a recognised fixed period, and in this way is fair to all. It might perhaps be argued that the retiring age should be different, that is *later* for those engaged in mental work. This is an illusion, and it is based on the idea that those who are doing primarily mental work have a longer spell of useful activity. But on the road of life the twilight is a treacherous time, because one of the most common early changes in mental capacity is the growing want of self-judgment. When we hear an elderly man saying that he is as good as ever he was, we can be fairly sure that he has begun to deteriorate in judgment, and is raising artificial defences. This is just like the old man who complains that young people do not speak clearly nowadays.

The portrait of a man or woman at the retiring age varies enormously from one country to another. It is often associated with the historical background of the country itself and the attitude of the people to its elders. On the one hand there are countries in which we have the drab picture of a man for whom no provision has been made. He has no outside interests and his retirement leads only to a desert of loneliness. In some of the older countries, on the other hand, the aged wield an almost uncanny authority and are looked up to as though all wisdom flowed from them. It is remarkable indeed at the present time how many countries are in the hands of aged people who in ordinary life would be retired and inactive.

The study of ageing is of practical and urgent value throughout the world. In the medical field good progress has been made by the demonstration that many crippled and even bedridden folk can be put on their feet and helped to live useful lives. At the same time we should direct our attention in the public health services to the prevention of disability or at least to postponement of the wearing-out process. As pension schemes increase in the various countries now provided with social services there is, in many cases, a great decline in the importance of men over sixty. With adequate schemes of this kind there is less incentive on the part of employers to look beyond the retiring age and find suitable jobs, or adjust certain processes or functions in an industry, to suit the slower pace of the elderly worker. Two things are needed: to find and use some method of assessing the mental and physical capacity of workers some time before they reach the retiring age; and to find or devise jobs for those who show continuing capacity of a kind normally to be absorbed into the everyday routines of industry.

The essentials of a good retirement job are that:

1. it should be paid;

2. it should be either on a part-time basis or lighter in the sense of reducing physical or mental strain, or—what is more important—slowing the pace;

3. it should be on a mental level not substantially less than the previous work—it is bad policy to draft intelligent men and women to inferior duties which give them no real satisfaction;

4. the worker should be prepared to co-operate in simple and effective tests of his mental and physical capacities and, if necessary, undergo a course of training for his new employment.

The selection of elderly people for new work should be based upon positive capacities and not on a negative list of dreary disabilities.

If the question of retirement were merely a matter of physical strength there would be little room for argument; but just as the child has special characteristics and aptitudes so also have the aged their individual features. We should look at the matter positively and interest should be directed towards discovering what each man or woman approaching pensionable age can still do well—perhaps better than his juniors. In all these cases, however, the man himself must not be the arbiter. He must learn to accept the dispassionate, independent assessment of his physical capacities, or we shall make no real progress towards finding suitable jobs for those who are on the threshold of old age. No country or authority can profit by having swarms of elderly advisers whose minds are likely to be fixed on the past. It would be a good plan to establish Youth Employment Officers for those who are entering their second youth.

One of the mistakes which are frequently made in the study of the capacities of the elderly is due to failure to distinguish between the threshold of age—or the first period of retirement—and true old age. Yet there are usually differences between these two periods as striking as those between the pre-school child and the child of school age. At the threshold the essential problem is to decide what kind of further work would be suitable for the retiring person, and whether he is physically fit to undertake it. It would have been better to use the term 'medically fit' to show that the threshold examination would include the usual tests of general fitness. At the later age different considerations begin to shape, and they become more prominent as age advances beyond, say, seventy-five years. At the latter time the main question is not fitness for remunerative employment in the strict sense, but rather some form of occupation which will maintain interest and give the elder a sense of being wanted. The needs of the elderly professional man or woman are clear enough, and those of the manual worker are not unlike:

Relaxation from the strain of full-time work. It is essential to move softly on the downward slope.

A job of similar quality and content to previous work, requiring for its performance some of the experience and judgment already acquired.

A job that is essentially more appropriate for elderly people than for the young—more sedentary, for example, and requiring less physical effort.

The job should not be paced for the younger man; it should be capable of adaptation to the slower rate of the aged. Precisely the same considerations apply to the physically handicapped.

The work for the old ought not to be a part-time continuation of the previous employment. The classification should be made on merit, and the candidate should on no account be placed in a position in which his work is liable to come into conflict with that of his successor.

I recently discussed this question with my colleague, Dr. Blyth Brooke, who has done so much for the employment of the older group. Dr. Blyth Brooke gave me a few notes, and these I now repeat; they are based on long and successful experience:

The principles underlying the operation of the Finsbury Employment Scheme are based on preserving as long as possible the physical and mental health of the aged by

1. giving them, in consequence of becoming wage-earners, an enhanced status in their own estimation, and in that of their neighbours;

2. allowing them, by virtue of doing useful work, to occupy a definite place in community life, instead of being outside its pale, as they so often are;

3. fulfilling for them a sub-conscious urge that most of us possess, to be of some service to mankind in our life;

4. proving to them that they are still wanted by others, and

5. providing for them a purpose in life.

It may be noted that, in effecting these ends, the personal obligations entailed in working are just as important as the privileges secured. These purposes overlap to a considerable extent, but taken together they add up to *self-respect*, which operates as a stimulus to give hope and to retain the wish to go on living.

There are certain subsidiary values in the scheme such as

1. the bodily and mental exercise necessary for dressing neatly and maintaining cleanliness in order to attend the workshop, going to work and carrying it out in the presence of others. Such matters tend to prevent a kind of disuse atrophy from complicating ordinary senescence;

2. the concern for their welfare shown by the Organiser, and often her affection—a great comfort for those who yearn for love;

3. the opportunity for companionship of fellow-workers in otherwise lonely lives;

4. the means of passing the time for those whose days seem very long, which is readily provided even by part-time employment; and last, and probably also least

5. the few extra moneys the elderly are able to earn, which allows those with very small incomes to obtain a little 'pocket-money' of their own, and so get something more than they would otherwise have or could afford.[12]

I should like to add a few explanations to show more exactly how the scheme fits in with other plans for the employment of the elderly. In the first place, it is in no sense an employment scheme for those who are on the threshold of age. It is intended for the old. It follows from this that the kind of employment no longer requires formal association with previous work. The chief object is to arouse and maintain interest among those who are tending to lose touch with life, and are falling into lonely desolation. The scheme aimed at providing employment for part of each day in congenial surroundings. The actual work hours are *either* from 9.45 to 11.45 *or* from 1.45 to 3.45. The work is provided mainly by local manufacturers as 'hand-outs'. The following are examples:

1. Outwork on behalf of commercial firms:
    (*a*) making elastic attachments for finger stalls.
    (*b*) assembling elements for electric irons.
    (*c*) assembling drop bottles for eyes, ears and throat.
    (*d*) weighing and packing animal wool for surgical purposes.
2. For direct sale, either wholesale or retail:
    (*a*) Coverings for coathangers.
    (*b*) making or decorating aprons.
    (*c*) making various nylon articles of dress.

The ordinary commercial rate is charged for outwork undertaken and goods made are sold privately or to business houses at fair rates. It should of course be noted that this work can be done effectively only through the willing and helpful co-operation of commercial firms.

In the financial year 1959-60 the loss was around 30 per cent, the difference being made good by voluntary subscriptions and contributions from the local council.

It is noteworthy that a very large number of schemes have been prepared and set in motion to deal with the employment of the aged; but comparatively few of these have shown any keen discrimination between the younger and the older group of ageing persons or have been able to transfer their clients from the active to the passive group as age advanced. Yet the distinction is real and important. The chief characteristic of the older group is that employment as such should be of a routine type, not demanding special skill or interest. The mere use of time is the essential, as it is sufficient to make the ageing person feel that he is of some use, and above all, it prevents the appalling sense of loneliness. For this reason simple employments of a routine character are desirable, such as the repetitive tasks of fitting things together, of inserting 'instructions' into packages, of closing small packages and sticking on the outer label. The workers should take their own time and should not be subject to a sense of rush; and they should be encouraged to talk to their neighbours. In fine, what is being advocated is suitable pay for entrants into second childhood. There is no need for the work to be wholly sedentary, so long as it does not involve any heavy lifting or the like. In other words, the key to the needs of this period is an understanding of childhood; and it is not without interest to learn that some of those who were first in the field in geriatrics, like Jacobi, were themselves pediatricians.

To sum up, there are two periods of ageing which should be recognised and differentiated. The first might well be called 'the threshold of age'. Its features at the present time are that the individual has been in some way discharged from his regular employment at a time when he is still fit to make a useful contribution to the community, although probably not in his old job. This age group ranges from 65 to 75, with a wide margin on both sides. On the other hand some grow old before their time, perhaps as a result of sickness; and some lose their employment at a fixed age, generally around 65. At the other extreme there are a substantial number who retain their activities far beyond the 'fixed age', and make great contributions to their community, their country, and even to the world. In terms of the ordinary worker, however, we are concerned to offer the first group an opportunity for continued useful, remunerative work although commonly at a slower pace and under less pressure than in their previous employment, whether mentally or physically.

REFERENCES

[1] PLATO Republic, Bk. I.
[2] JOHNSON, SAMUEL, The Rambler
[3] BACON, Essays, XLII.
[4] TENNYSON, Ulysses.
[5] BROWNING, Rabbi ben Ezra.
[6] HARDY, An Ancient to Ancients.
[7] MARTIN, LILIAN J. & DE GRUCHY, CLARE, (1960): Salvaging Old Age, New York, Macmillan.
[8] Joint Report on the Public Assistance Institutions of Northampton, 1930.
[9] LATHROP, REV. S. G. (1881): Fifty Years and Beyond, New York, Revell.
[10] KUTNER, BERNARD, et al. (1956): Five Hundred Over Sixty: A Community Survey of Aging; Russell Sage Foundation, New York (Association of New York City Health Department and Cornell Medical College and Social Science Research Center).
[11] Annual Report, 1911.
[12] BROOKE, C. BLYTH, The Finsbury (London) Employment Scheme for the Elderly.

Chapter 13

ACCIDENTS AS A WORLD PROBLEM

The study of the prevention of accidents as a world problem rests on three pillars. The first of these is *legislation,* that is, the prescription of definite measures to promote safety and to protect people from hazards which can be foreseen. The second may be described as *epidemiology,* that is, the study of facts in relation to accidental injuries and deaths; without knowledge of the extent and the changing incidence of accidents in each country, it would not be possible to forecast even the legal requirements. And thirdly, there is *education,* that is, the deliberate teaching and training of children by practice and example to understand the risks and to know what action should be taken to avoid them.

Many other features can be considered as part of the intricate scheme of prevention. This applies, for example, to the actual provision of emergency treatment for accidental injuries. This immediate action may make all the difference between recovery and serious crippling, or even loss of life. In this growing and important development first aid, as it is called, takes a prominent part. It is the vanguard activity, and is particularly valuable because it can be taught to lay people, and even to children at a relatively early age of responsibility. The second aspect is the provision of adequate skilled emergency treatment through the establishment of clinics, accident centres, and special hospital units. This has been an important advance during the past decade in a number of countries, as well as in industry. One of the essential features of the programme of emergency care is to have means of dealing with the exact type of accident which is likely to occur in a given situation. Submersion, poisoning and burning accidents are among the dangers that demand special and skilled attention. In addition, the rising toll of traffic accidents has created a new type of treatment centre in which special attention has to be paid to the prevention of shock and to the restoration of blood volume. In the more highly developed areas, this demand has created a modern type of 'accident treatment centre', which is open day and night all the year round, and which is staffed by nursing and medical personnel capable of dealing with any kind of emergency.

The approach to the world problem would be grossly incomplete without reference to the modern conception of *disaster planning* on a large scale. This organisation has been developed extensively by the Red Cross and by co-operative hospital groups, especially in the United States; but the idea is applicable to every part of the world. It is the first line of defence against the vagaries of nature—earthquake, flood, fire and tempest—and man's inhumanity to man as represented by the shock of war, the plight of refugees and the homeless. Disaster planning is also a bulwark of strength in the greater accident situations, such as rail and air disasters, extensive fires, and traffic catastrophes such as occur all too frequently on the more recently constructed highways. In this preventive work, teams of helpers have to be prepared and carefully trained in co-operation. Plans have to be drawn up to ensure that sufficient assistance is always at hand, generally based on hospitals, and that organisations over a large area can be alerted from a central source at short notice. Without keen and regular practice between one area and another any scheme is likely itself to end in disaster: the readiness is all.

The emergency aspects of medical care, and especially first aid and teamwork, is of the utmost importance to preventive medicine throughout the world, and should be extended as part of the essential equipment of every advance in industrial and urban development. But this does not get to the root of the accident problem, nor does it go very far towards satisfying the needs of countries which are now on the threshold of industrial and social advance. It is clear enough that the best time to deal with an accident successfully is before it happens, and as a result of this one must lay greater stress on the forward planning than on dealing with the emergency as it arises.

THE CONTRIBUTION OF LAW TO PREVENTION

Recognition of the outstanding place to be taken by accidents as a cause of sickness and death has been remarkably slow. This is partly due to the failure in many of the developing countries to appreciate the value of legal measures, taken in advance, as the prime agent in prevention. It is true that accounts of accidental happenings, including the effects of supernatural forces, have appeared many times in the literature of the world, and indeed the legal expression 'an act of God' survives to this day and has been defined as 'an act which no reasonable man would expect'. The accident situation first appeared as an ugly prominence in the world over a century ago, in the countries which were then making rapid strides in industrial development. At that time the toll of death and injury among children alone in factories and workplaces was very heavy, and much of it preventable. In the course of the nineteenth century, especially in Germany, legislation was gradually introduced to limit, and ultimately to prohibit, the employment of women and children in factories where dangerous processes were being carried out, and in several countries of Europe the employment of children in factories was prohibited and great strides were made in protecting the worker generally from dangerous processes and ill-designed machinery. In spite of the difficulties of enforcement, the grip of the law gradually extended towards the small workshop and the home, where the worst industrial conditions were often found. Today, most of the industrial countries possess a comprehensive code of legislation providing for health and safety, much of which could be applied with only minor modifications, to any industrially advancing country in the world.

Again, the enormous development of road traffic since the beginning of the present century has brought to the fore the dramatic role of accidents as a world problem. Although furious driving was mentioned in ancient Hebrew literature, the situation did not achieve notoriety until the twentieth century, even in countries where mechanical transport had become considerable. In England a number of important legal decisions had been taken over a century ago. In the year 1841 a Mr. Davies fettered the forefeet of his donkey and turned the animal loose on the public highway. This in itself was an illegal act under the common law. Shortly afterwards, a Mr. Mann, driving his horse and wagon, as he admitted, 'at a smartish pace', ran over and killed the donkey. On appeal,

Mann was held liable because, by taking ordinary care, he could have avoided the consequences of the plaintiff's negligence. This famous leading case was the foundation of the law of contributory negligence. Nearly a quarter of a century later the legal position was further clarified by what is known as the Rule in Rylands v. Fletcher. This runs roughly as follows: a person who for his own purposes keeps anything likely to do mischief if it escapes, must keep it at his peril and, if it does break loose, is answerable for all the consequences. Actually the original case was not a tiger, but the escape of water down a mineshaft which had not been noticed during the construction of a reservoir. In some European countries, however, the law is still moving slowly towards the doctrine of special responsibility in the case of accidents. For example, the theory of objective responsibility has now been extended to a legal presumption of offence against a driver in the case of an innocent pedestrian, unless he can prove specifically that he is not liable.

ROAD TRAFFIC AND THE LAW TODAY

In recent years, during which automobile traffic has become a common-place all over the world, the number of road accidents has risen in a baleful partnership with the increase in the number of vehicles. Health officers make reference to various preventive aspects, notably through educational and general safety measures. Their task is also to point out the value of law as a preventive agent, especially in countries which are being faced with this situation for the first time. In these areas, even before the dawn of intelligent traffic control, a vigorous policy of positive regulation by means of town and country planning and the proper location of industry, could do a great deal to prevent the slaughter on the roads. The foundations of good planning are law and order.

First in time and importance come the technical prescriptions which are readily enforceable. Those concerned with traffic include precise regulations dealing with the construction of roads, railways and other channels of transport. Among these may be mentioned the capacity of bridges to withstand the violence of nature in flood and tempest; the stability of structural work on surfaces and cuttings; and measures for the protection of children at road and rail crossings. The point of greatest danger is the cross road in both town and country, and the proper time to provide security is while the road is being built. At the planning stage, important crossings should be left open and free from buildings, so that under-passes can be constructed even before the traffic conditions justify the cost.

In plans for the traffic of the future, the great arterial roads must be regarded as on the same plane as the railroads of the past, and it will be necessary to introduce a special signalling system if multiple collisions are to be avoided. In other words, careful studies ought to be made of preventive measures *before* a great highway system is put into operation, and not after it has been strewn with bodies. A simple case in point is the three-lane road, which has turned out to be a death-trap. In modern road construction it will soon be declared illegal. However, this is an exact illustration of the importance of planning as a preventive measure.

LEGAL PRESCRIPTIONS DEALING WITH FIXED STRUCTURES AND INSTALLATIONS

In the homes of the people, especially in the less developed countries, there are limits to what the law can do. Nevertheless, experience has built up a valuable series of regulations relating to the safety of buildings as structures: the strength of their foundations, the minimum height of rooms, and the safe load of walls and roofs. The materials used in construction should be required to pass certain tests, especially for safety and fire-resistance. The protection of the child at play against traps and hazards of every kind has to be assured by regulation, and not left to chance, as is happening in too many areas of the world at the present time. In the more advanced countries special prescriptions are gradually being introduced to cover the layout, construction and safety of temporary buildings—which have proved themselves to be a grave risk even when they are wholly on the ground floor. Unhappily, in some of the rapidly developing towns and suburban areas, where the inrush of population in search of work is considerable, too little forward planning is being carried out, with the result that the dwellings of the workers are scrambled together and are positively dangerous to health and safety. The shanty town is still with us, and the negligence of today will be the vain regret of tomorrow.

Admittedly, some of the regulations which can be properly applied to industry are too restrictive to the informal conditions of the home. There is also the obvious difficulty of enforcing or even supervising the regulation of the home. In spite of this, precise rules have an important place in the protection of children in their homes, so long as the rules are in line with the traditions of the people and hold their confidence. Strict provisions can be made, for example, in the manufacture of toys, in the prohibition of dangerous substances such as lead in the composition of paint, or highly flammable material in children's clothing. In the same way, rules can be widely enforced for the protection of children against harmful drugs or materials used around the home in cleaning, or as fuel. Of course the best laid schemes for safety can be wantonly destroyed by the negligence of parents or other guardians of the young child.

Provision against the risk of fire includes, as a legal requirement which ought to be on a world scale, minimum standards of safety construction and effective means of escape from all floors of a building, irrespective of the use of lifts. Up to the present, far too little attention has been paid to safety exits from public buildings and large blocks of flats, and to the essential provision of doors that open outwards on simple pressure from the inside. Similarly, the prescription of a maximum and minimum width for staircases and the compulsory provision of handrails are important measures of safety, especially in schools, cinemas and other public buildings. The reason for the maximum width is the danger of a panic rush overwhelming children and weaker members of the public who might otherwise be able to move to the side of the stairway quite easily. The wider the stair, the greater the danger.

CODES OF CONDUCT FOR INDIVIDUALS AND GROUPS

On the roads and elsewhere the demands of the law must be reasonable and well adapted to the level of education and understanding of the people in whose interests they are applied. It is of the utmost importance that rules having the force of law should not be allowed to fall into desuetude. The best-marked pedestrian crossings are dangerous in some European countries because they are persistently overlooked by police and ignored by drivers. It is pitiful to watch frightened pedestrians having to scuttle across crossings that were marked for their benefit, but only serve as an additional hazard. On the other hand, legal enforcement should not try to exercise greater power than is needed to achieve a particular end. It is better to have a few rules, universally observed, than a multitude of complex signs and regulations that cause annoyance and invite disobedience. The proper function of legal measures should be considered against the background of custom, tradition and educational level in each country. It has to be remembered that the making of rules comes *before* their acceptance by any community, and that in the advancing countries preventive regulations will secure conditions from the start that were reached in the older communities only after great distress and a heavy record of injury and death. Even young children can undoubtedly be trained to observe traffic signs if they are reasonably simple and uniform in size and colour for each type of indication, and if the legal requirements carry the confidence and support of the great majority of citizens, but the child cannot be trained to observe signals which are not there!

Epidemiology on the World Scale

Epidemiology is one of the foundations of accident prevention because facts are the basis of action. Accurate knowledge permits the statistician to draw analogies between one country and another, especially when the general lines of progress are similar. In this respect, epidemiology must look at the trends rather than to the past and present. For example, a recent sample of a large region in Africa indicates that the chief accident problems of today are represented by falls from trees, drownings in rivers, snake-bites and injuries caused by wild animals; but the picture is changing rapidly and it would obviously be wrong to found preventive measures on the prevailing pattern of injury. Nevertheless, the study of comparative statistics will tell us a great deal about the direction and pace of the change, the effects of age and sex, and the realities that are likely to prevail. A careful study of patterns, usually on a sample basis, may readily disclose ways of prevention that will provide a short cut to what has hitherto been a long process of trial and error.

The increase in traffic hazards is only one of the problems to which urgent attention has to be directed in the developing countries. Other risks, such as those related to the sudden use of electricity, or radiation, in home and factory, and the steady increase in the use of economic poisons, may alter almost overnight the processes of industrial development, especially in a community which was previously largely agricultural. There is an element of urgency in accident prevention and in the employment of educational measures, which has not been felt until recent years. This is particularly true in countries where general education has lagged behind industrial advance.

In the highly industrialised countries also, the pattern of accidental injuries is apt to change abruptly. The decline in the use of open fires in England, for example, will reduce the incidence of burning accidents in the home, but at the same time the more extensive use of electricity in radio and television, and in many forms of domestic apparatus, offers too much scope to the amateur electrician. In the United States especially, the widespread use of self-medication, combined with the attractive wrappings of potentially dangerous drugs, has increased the hazard of poisoning in the home. In some cases, indeed, it is difficult for legislation to keep up with the ingenuity of the manufacturer of dangerous substances. In the older world of affairs many of these things are a commonplace, and their use has limited the risks, but this is not so in the developing countries, where the new materials and processes have come in with a rush, and often without the taking of essential precautions either by the dealer or by the local legislature. In addition, the lack of accurate figures and the want of statistical services in many of these areas tend to delay preventive measures until the danger has reached large dimensions.

EDUCATIONAL BASIS

One of the difficulties in dealing with the prevention of accidents from the educational point of view is to decide at what age teaching should begin. The education of boys and girls from the age of twelve or so is probably the most effective way of reaching the minds of prospective parents. It is also a time when imaginative teaching is intelligently absorbed, and when many of the duties of parenthood can be learned simply as part of the ordinary process of acquiring knowledge. One of the subjects on which research is needed is the best way of approach to children of early adolescent age. If, for example, the parents themselves live carelessly, the young children are unconsciously exposed to danger. In the same way the influence of the immediate surroundings on parent and child is very strong. It is essential at first to remove from a child's environment those things which create a hazard to life. Parents may expose themselves to danger without realising that in so doing they are exposing their children to an even greater risk. There are not a few cases in which people deliberately and light-heartedly encourage children to court danger. This incitement is to be deprecated, and every effort should be made to convince the public that when parents and officials take protective action they should be supported by all, because their main consideration is safety.

If we take the phases of childhood from the beginning, accidents in the first years of life are limited to a great extent by the helplessness of the baby. Many simple precautions are thought of as instinctive in the young mother, but on the whole it is better to rely on training and practice during pregnancy and early maternity than to face unnecessary risks. This is one of the great advantages of group training, which can be so effectively given in infant welfare centres. It is there that the anxious mother often has her fears stilled by contact with a more robust group, and especially with those who have already had experience of bringing up children. There is nothing so effective as the exchange of actual experience between the mothers, always provided that this takes place under some kind of skilled supervision, for example, that of the public health nurse. In addition to group teaching, the nurse can do a great deal through her home visits. By even a superficial look around the house she is able to point out any special risks relating to furniture, fittings, flooring and stairways, and she can take the opportunity of watching the mother during the preparation of meals and tactfully point out the dangers and show how they can be avoided. This applies especially to the habit of laying utensils like kettles and saucepans on the floor, or on a stove with their handles projecting, and many other careless habits of this kind. Giving advice on the care of the baby in the home offers an opportunity of teaching how to prepare a bath for the baby, and the obvious risks of putting in the hot water first, or leaving a jug of hot water where there is a child of pre-school age in the vicinity. All these difficulties are of course enhanced when the kitchen is small or when cooking has to be done in the living room.

When the child is active enough to reach the crawling stage, he requires a great deal of personal attention, and the mother's function is to keep dangerous articles out of reach, while at the same time giving him as much free play as possible. These situations are commonplace enough, but they point the way to positive teaching of simple precautions.

The third stage of growth in childhood is the pre-school period, during which greatly increased activity and opportunity for exploration leads a child into quite a different series of hazards. Special care must be taken by both parents to keep dangerous articles out of reach. The father now carries an extra responsibility, especially if he is inclined towards amateur carpentry and electrical work. The danger runs to gas taps, water and baths, and more particularly to electrical fittings such as radio and television. Parents cannot escape responsibility for these, because they have a duty to make sure that the contents of the house are reasonably safe, or in case of doubt to obtain the services of an expert to advise them. At the present time there are not enough arrangements for expert supervision of people's homes, although an increasing number of local authorities undertake housing responsibilities. During this period a great deal can be done by direct teaching of the child, and the natural guide is the parent. Frequently, however, the parents themselves need to be taught how to get it across to the wayward child. It has even been suggested by some that the best safety device is actual experience. This is a dangerous guide in inexpert hands. The deliberate use of trial by injury may lead a sensitive child towards distrust of his parents—a position which it will be hard to alter in later years. As a rule, the only reasonable solution is deliberate teaching of the mother by the public health nurse, by demonstrations and exhibits, by health authorities and voluntary organisations interested in protection. It is important in everyday teaching to bring safety into line with ordinary advice and guidance, and not to lay undue emphasis on the risk of injury. In other words, teaching—especially to children—should be positive in the sense of showing safety precautions rather than the results of injury. Some recent posters give both sides of the question and may confuse the minds of children and make them experiment with what has been intended as a caution.

As the child reaches school age, the emphasis of teaching ought to shift from the parents to stimulating the child's own sense of responsibility. He should be given the suggestion that he himself is able to accept a position of trust, and teaching for children of the younger ages ought to concentrate on self-reliance. Although the parents are primarily responsible for safety, they ought to have a powerful ally in the teacher. Simple home training in the family should be supplemented by more detailed application in the school. This applies especially to safety rules and practice in traffic, and instruction later on in both protection and first aid, particularly in swimming and preventing injuries in connection with bicycles, etc. If no teaching has been given in the home, the teacher's task is all the more difficult because one of the most impressionable ages has already been passed. Prevention is a consciously planned activity. If teachers are to do their work for the promotion of safety, they must themselves be taught, so that instruction to teachers-in-training is not served by casual reference to accidents during the educational curriculum. It requires all the concentration of a special course of training, both theoretical and practical. A subject of such importance to the children cannot be left to the odd lecture or demonstration, even when that is given by a specially trained teacher. A course of training for student teachers is inescapable, and it is best undertaken by one of the staff specially trained in this subject, or by a voluntary organisation. The essential function of such a course is training in *how to teach children*, and not merely accident prevention and the value of safety measures.

At the same time, it should not be thought that a general course of teaching would be satisfactory. Preventive agencies, for example, the Red Cross, become highly specialised in dealing with a single subject such as drowning or poisoning, and so it is desirable to arrange courses which bring in specialists in these particular subjects; and excellent pioneer work in fact has been done in this respect by the Red Cross, using films and demonstrations.

The brief account of educational methods which has been given above lays its emphasis deliberately on the value of simplicity. This applies with greatly increased force to the less developed areas of the world. It is the simple message that strikes home; the complex only confuses, and the results are often disastrous. A second feature of teaching which is effective throughout the world as a means of accident prevention is the value of repetition, preferably in forms which enable variation in detail to maintain the interest of the audience and to lead to positive action. It can be clearly shown, however, that an educational method, even when expressed with great ingenuity by voice and illustration, is not sufficient. It must be accompanied by action in which those taught take an intelligent part. Sensible precautions become a routine only after they have been applied over and over again, and this important fact should be realised in the simpler educational methods employed in the less developed countries. Learning by doing is the right approach, and plans in which the learner has some responsibility are always the best. It is difficult to visualise information by speech or writing, especially when children are in question. One of the first efforts should therefore be to set up a properly designed demonstration and to encourage parents, as well as their children, to visit it. This approach has been made effectively in a number of countries as a means of dealing with traffic risks. In Finland, for example, education for the prevention of accidents on the road is emphasised by providing in the parks a 'safety playground'. In this, the children themselves act as policemen, passengers and traffic controllers. Other children drive in toy cars, and the whole system of traffic control is learned by the use of signs and safety slogans.

The idea of demonstration as a forewarning is just as sound in and around the home, although the actual demonstration may be given in a school or some other public place. It is in its essence a method of training in social responsibility, which parents can follow up in the home and teachers in the school.

In some of the fully developed communities it is argued with a good deal of force that people tend to overprotect their children, and to give them too little responsibility. One effect of this might well be the reverse of what is aimed at, in making them more prone to accidents. For example, in some of the simpler societies children do perfectly well when they are left alone to find out many of the hazards for themselves, and they adapt themselves better in this 'school of experience'. This is no doubt true in communities where the number of possible dangers is small and the ways of avoiding these dangers are universally recognised and practised by all in the presence of the children. In simple village life the open fire, the oil lamp or candle, the bucket and the well, and the care of more or less domesticated animals are fully understood as part of the direct process of learning how to live. Nevertheless, statistical analysis shows unmistakably that even in the remote communities with few external associations, the casualty risk is greater than had been expected. Examples can be multiplied: the uncovered wells of Norway, the unprotected lakes and coasts of the Scandinavian countries, and the disastrous effects of extreme cold and heat in different climates. Good education as a preventive measure lies in the realm between over-casualness on the one hand and careless neglect on the other. We need facts in place of assumptions; well planned education in contrast to happy-go-lucky attitudes.

The real world problem of tomorrow has to be examined in the new light of technical advances. It is not primarily the under-developed communities that should be concerned with the question of education in accident prevention, but those which are entering industrial competition for the first time. It is not the status of the country that should cause anxiety, but the period of change upon which it is about to enter. A static community has, of course, problems of its own, but the rapidly developing community emerging tomorrow from its village life into the perils of industrial competition is a different story. But it must be told; and education must be concerned mainly with the hazards on the very threshold of economic and industrial advance. In the more prosperous industrial areas which have been planned around special resources such as oil wells, or newly discovered treasures underground, or it may be a labour force working on hydro-electric power stations in hitherto undeveloped areas—in these it may be anticipated that modern equipment will have been supplied or at least made accessible. Even in the well planned district the new hazards are bound to be considerable. But where industrial life has been introduced, as in certain parts of Africa, without the courtesy of design, the situation is likely to be positively dangerous. It would be grossly unfair to expect education to make good deficiencies to this extent. Yet it must do what it can, even against fearful odds. In many ways the situation is even worse when urbanization is taking place in the absence of new sources of employment, and the industrial shanty town is replaced by terrible overcrowding of already insufficient and insanitary habitations. In this case, however, the greater danger is sickness, rather than accident; sordid poverty and the ills that neither health campaigns nor legislation can materially diminish.

Chapter 14

DAMAGE IN THE NEW TOWNS

> One point must still be greatly dark,
> The moving *Why* they do it;
> And just as lamely can ye mark,
> How far perhaps they rue it.
>
> Then at the balance let's be mute,
> *We* never can adjust it;
> What's done we partly may compute,
> But know not what's resisted.
>
> (Robert Burns: Address to the Unco Guid)

This report on damage in the New Towns was based on an enquiry carried out under a grant from the Nuffield Foundation. Much of the detailed work of visiting and reporting was done with the assistance of Miss Gillian Beath, whose help was invaluable, both in investigation and in organization of the findings. Since the report was completed, we have made considerable studies of the more recently built estates associated with older communities, by way of comparison with the New Towns, and much more information has been received from other countries by correspondence and visiting—particularly in the United States and in Europe.

In view of housing plans recently put forward in England and elsewhere, which include the construction of a further group of New Towns, studies of this kind have acquired a new urgency, and we have received encouragement from the Nuffield Foundation to devote further attention to a number of the problems of today. These have been included in the present report.

The first object of our original enquiry was to confirm the facts by personal investigation. On our visits to the New Towns in England and Scotland we enjoyed the cordial co-operation of the staff of the Corporations, school teachers, general practitioners, health visitors and other workers who have access to the homes of the people in the course of their everyday duties. We relied on personal interviews with the tenants rather than on formal questionnaire, and we should like to express our gratitude to all those who gave so freely of their time and experience.

At an early stage we came to the conclusion that it would be valuable to make a number of additional investigations into the position on new estates built in well established communities. We felt that they would serve as a useful comparison with the New Towns, and also with estates of many years standing. It was interesting to find, for example, at what point in their history new communities began to be stabilized, and whether a reduction in the extent of damage was a feature of stabilization. Accordingly we enlarged our plan and subsequently made many visits to estates set up by local housing authorities throughout the country. In this work also we received great assistance from members of the staffs of local authorities and from social workers engaged in research in similar fields.

The third subject which we took up as a result of our experience in the field was to analyze our findings and to suggest measures which might be taken to prevent wanton and malicious damage. As a result of this study we made a number of recommendations. Many of these were chiefly concerned with following up by further experiment some of the ideas raised in our original enquiry. We also had the benefit, as time went on, from other studies of parallel subjects, and we carried on a large international correspondence.

The original enquiry was undertaken in 1957 and 1958 and the report which we prepared at that time was transmitted to the various authorities responsible for the development of New Towns. The following essay is based on this report, but we have gained the benefit of further studies by other investigators, as well as our own reconsideration of the major problems involved.

CHARACTERISTICS OF NEW TOWNS AND ESTATES

The aim of policy in building the New Towns in Britain was to provide homes for the surplus populations of cities: to provide them in self-contained communities separated from existing urban development by preserving as far as possible 'green belts' in which no building is allowed. The distinguishing feature of the New Towns is that factories as well as people are encouraged to move in. It is the combination of home and place of work that makes a real community. The New Towns are therefore inhabited in the main by enterprising couples with young families. There are few old folk, and the adolescents were at first in no great number.

In the new estates developed by older communities the position is somewhat different. Some of these estates have been built as a means to slum clearance, and there has been an inevitable measure of compulsion in the transfer. The housing authorities do not always appreciate that the tenants coming from clearance areas may suffer a double handicap—an element of pressure to secure their removal and the fact that rehousing does not necessarily carry with it the provision of suitable employment. One result of this experience is that the tenants from clearance areas have less incentive than the other group to regard the new estate as their permanent home, and many sigh for the attractions of the old locality. In such circumstances one would expect to find more damage, careless or deliberate, on the 'clearance estates'. This is probably true, but the matter is complicated by the fact that, when such families are brought out to the fringe of well-established districts, there are often exaggerated complaints of destruction and bad behaviour on the part of the newcomers. No doubt matters settle down in the course of time, but there is sometimes a lingering hostility.

We must not exaggerate the seriousness of our problem, or give the false impression that wanton damage by a youth places him on the threshold of delinquency. Boys, and even girls, have always been known to indulge in all manner of mischief for its own sake, but are not on that account to be labelled as patients with problems of behaviour. The good parent and the good teacher recognize these difficulties and surmount most of them by the exercise of patience and common sense. A good home and a good school lead children to a normal and happy adult life, provided always that there is a close and sympathetic understanding between home and school.

Many detailed researches of great value have been carried out on the delinquent child and the adolescent gang. Much has been written also about the educationally sub-normal, and the maladjusted. The histories of deprived children have been carefully examined and documented, and studies of 'problem families' have revealed much that is of prime importance to the mental health of parents and children. The subject of this essay, however, is the 'ordinary' child.

A NOTE ON HISTORY

THE CITY OF THE ANCIENT WORLD

In their brilliant and sombre book, The Age of the Chartists, the Hammonds contrast the cities of the ancient world with the new towns of the industrial revolution in Great Britain. In doing so they try to discover a difference between the concepts of government in Graeco-Roman civilization and in nineteenth century England. The struggles between rich and poor in ancient Greece were bitter and lawless, and the rioting mobs of the latter days of the Roman Republic were no doubt more ferocious and cruel than those of eighteenth century England, when 'a licentious, riotous, seditious, and almost ungovernable spirit in the people showed itself in many tumults and disorders in different shapes and in different parts of the kingdom'.[1] But in the first half of the nineteenth century we are more struck by the silence and deep resentment of the working people than by the noise of rioting and destruction.

So long as we remember that these ancient civilizations were supported by slavery which was officially recognized, the explanation put forward by the Hammonds is convincing and relevant to this essay. It amounts briefly to this: that in the many varieties of political government an effort was made to command the wills of men, and not merely their deeds and services. 'The class struggle was veiled or softened by the moral influence of common possessions; the practice of social fellowship was stimulated by the spectacle of beautiful buildings, and the common enjoyment of the arts and culture of the time.'[2] It was for this reason that the mutilation of the statues, attributed to Alcibiades as leader of a gang, was so shocking to Athenian public opinion. In the same way the secret of the power and stability of the Roman Empire was its genius in satisfying the peoples which came under its rule. A great part of its wealth was devoted to buildings and amenities designed for common enjoyment. Every city had its public games and festivals, its theatres and its public baths, and above all, the great gardens and parks for relaxation and amusement. Julius Caesar was following, in his generous fashion, the tradition of the age, when he left to the people

> All his walks,
> His private arbours, and new-planted orchards,
> On this side Tiber; he hath left them you,
> And to your heirs for ever—common pleasures,
> To walk abroad, and recreate yourselves.

. . . and the people responded as they would today, as in Shakespeare's time, in revenge for his murder:

> 2nd citizen: Go fetch fire.
> 3rd citizen: Pluck down benches.
> 4th citizen: Pluck down forms, windows, any thing.

The New Town of the Nineteenth Century

In the new town of the nineteenth century the position of the people was the reverse of what is happening today. The industrial town was busy absorbing the rural worker used to the open-air life, to the peace and slow movement of the country. It was moulding him to the hard, impersonal routine of the factory, and to a sunless life in slum streets and alleys. Another sinister feature of the change was that in these new towns there was no provision for common enjoyment. Wealth and its showings were owned by private persons, and there were few festivals or amusements to bring people together. Libraries and museums, public parks and pleasure grounds, theatres and music halls had no place in the new town. The success and wealth of private individuals supplanted the idea of common enjoyment.

During the first half of the nineteenth century England could boast of only one institution, the Poor Law, which was charged with the burdens of maintaining health and social welfare. It is therefore not surprising to find that the lay-out and construction of the new industrial towns was left in the hands of the speculative builder, unhampered by any rules of planning or regulations for design, decency, or even safety.

N

Many examples of the sordid consequences might be taken from the Reports of the Health of Towns Commission (1844) and other accounts of the period, but two selections will be enough to penetrate the gloom:

Of Liverpool it was reported that 'the soil is subdivided into a multitude of holdings, and a man runs a new street, generally as narrow as he possibly can, through a field, not only to save the greater expense of soughing and paving, which, in the first instance, falls upon himself, but also that he may have a greater quantity of land to dispose of. The next owner continues that street, if it suits him, but he is not obliged to do so, and the consequence is the growth of narrow thoroughfares, the erection of mean edifices, the utter neglect of proper sewerage, the in-attention to ventilation, and that train of evils which is so much to be deplored. . .

Again, of Manchester, 'An immense number of small houses occupied by the poorer classes in the suburbs are of the most superficial character; they are built by the members of building clubs, and other individuals, and new cottages are erected with a rapidity that astonishes persons who are unacquainted with their flimsy structure. They have certainly avoided the objectionable mode of forming underground dwellings, but have run into the opposite extreme, having neither cellar nor foundation. The walls are only half-brick thick, or what the bricklayers call 'brick noggin', and the whole of the materials are slight and unfit for the purpose. They are built back-to-back, without ventilation or drainage; and, like a honeycomb, every particle of space is occupied. Double rows of these houses form courts, with, perhaps, a pump at one end and a privy at the other, common to the occupants of about twenty houses'.

Comments like this could be made of practically every industrial town of the time, and it has taken more than a century to remove the worst of the slum areas created in the days before planning was thought of, except by a few enlightened owners.

Loss of Playgrounds

From our point of view an equally tragic situation was created by the loss of public playgrounds, under the system of enclosures. A vivid description is given in the 1845 Report of the town of Basford, near Nottingham. As much as fifty years after the enclosures of 1793 the want of open land was still a source of gang warfare between the young men of the parish and the owners and occupiers of the land. There were frequent 'trespasses for cricket playing and other games'. The Hammonds give an interesting account of Blackburn, showing the actual deterioration of the position in the nineteenth century:

> In 1618 the 1266 acres of common and waste land were enclosed and divided up amongst the owners of land in Blackburn, but some 18 acres were to be set out and used for 'the mustering and training of people in that part, and for the recreation of the Inhabitants of the said Town and Poor thereof, as a gift for ever. . .' The rights of recreation had apparently been lost by 1833. 'Is there any place', William Feilden, M.P. for Blackburn, was then asked, 'to which the children of the humbler classes may resort for any game or exercise, any of those games they have been used to on holidays'? 'None whatever', was the answer.

In Birmingham, although there were no public parks or open spaces, a fair proportion of the people had gardens of their own. In giving evidence to the Committee on Public Walks in 1833, one of the Birmingham witnesses observed that the working men paid about a guinea a year and that a great many of the workers went there with their families: 'They have little summer houses where they spend their evenings and Sundays'. Within ten years it was reported that the gardens had all been built over, 'and the mechanics of this town are gradually losing this source of useful and healthy recreation'.

The lack of public parks tells the same dismal story: In 1833 Dr. J. P. Kay, in giving evidence to the Committee on Public Walks, wrote:

> At present the entire labouring population of Manchester is without any season of recreation, and is ignorant of all amusements, excepting that very small portion which frequents the theatres. Healthful exercise in the open air is seldom or never taken by the artisans of this town, and their health certainly suffers considerable depression from this deprivation. One reason of this state of the people is that all scenes of interest are remote from the town, and that the walks which can be enjoyed by the poor are chiefly the turnpike roads, alternately dusty or muddy. Were parks provided, recreation would be taken with avidity, and one of the first results would be a better use of the Sunday, and a substitution of innocent amusement at all other times, for the debasing pleasures now in vogue. I need not tell you how sad is our labouring population here.

It is pleasant to know that the plea for public parks was justified in the event, although that was long postponed. The opening of three parks, secured by public subscription, was a great occasion in 1846. There is no doubt whatever of the value of these parks and open spaces in terms of behaviour.

The first conference of the National Association for the Promotion of Social Science was held in 1858. One of the speakers gave a most illuminating report on a chapter of local history. In the town of Macclesfield, he explained, the death-rate in the year was 42 per thousand, and for this one undrained district of seven streets was responsible as well as for practically all the crime of the town. The Public Health Act of 1848 was adopted and the district was made sanitary. Within ten years the death-rate had fallen to 26 per thousand. Baths and wash-houses had been installed and a public park was purchased in which as many as 40 cricket matches were sometimes played on a single Saturday afternoon when the mills were closed. This park was filled with people every evening in summer and its opening was followed by a striking decrease in crime. The speaker[3] then quoted the following figures:

> The question might fairly be asked, what would become of the large masses of people who congregate in the park on a summer's evening after work if they had no such place of resort? The answer is in some measure suggested by a reference to the police records of the past. Since the opening of the park, cases of 'drunkenness and disorderly conduct' have decreased in the borough 23 per cent, as compared with the preceding three years. 'Making use of obscene and profane language' has decreased 60 per cent. Gambling has decreased 58 per cent; and summary charges of every class have decreased 26 per cent.

TOWN AND COUNTRY PLANNING

In England the apathy of Government, which delayed the provision of parks and open spaces for public recreation and permitted the creation of slums innumerable, was repeated on a smaller scale in the present century. The idea of the garden city was put forward by Ebenezer Howard in 1898, and Letchworth was built some four years later. In 1909 a feeble piece of planning legislation was introduced, with the usual effect of postponing action. At the close of the first world war the Government started a great drive towards housing, but showed little interest in town planning, and still less in garden cities. It was not until the evil of ribbon development had spread through the country like an eczema that the notion of planning was taken up once more, with the Act of 1932.

In spite of lack of encouragement, Howard set out upon a second venture in 1920, and the flourishing Welwyn Garden City was the result. It is interesting to note that a loan was eventually obtained for the Welwyn project from the Public Works Loan Commissioners under the provisions of a section of the Housing Act of 1921.

During the thirties the main interest of Parliament was very properly directed to slum clearance, and later to the mitigation of overcrowding. Town planning might well have gone along side by side, but it was dealt with piecemeal, and for the most part without imagination. In this period, as it happened, various conditions combined to put forward a policy for limiting the further growth of the great towns. A Royal Commission under the chairmanship of Sir Montagu Barlow was appointed in 1937 'to consider what social, economic or strategical disadvantages arise from the concentration of industries and of the industrial population in large towns or in particular areas of the country; and to report what remedial measures, if any, should be taken in the national interest'.

The Barlow Report put forward, as one of its main recommendations, a proposal for the creation of a new agency, independent of existing government departments, to collect the facts of the situation and to undertake research into the problem of redeveloping congested urban areas, and dispersing industries and population in such a way as to get a better balance of industrial townships throughout the country, combined of course with greater safety. Satellite towns, garden cities, and trading estates were mentioned, together with the enlargement of existing small towns. The Report led to a further enquiry on problems of dispersal (the Uthwatt Committee). These committees endorsed the Barlow recommendation to establish a new central authority. In ordinary circumstances these Reports might have been subject to prolonged controversies, but the sharp stimulus of war and destruction of cities led, as early as 1943, to the creation of a central authority—the Ministry of Town and Country

Planning.* Although little action in the field could be taken until the end of the war, steady preparatory work was undertaken by the new Ministry, for the control of development in the interim and for readier acquisition of land.

In the flood of legislation that followed the war special attention was given to the establishment of national parks and the preservation of rural amenities. In 1947 a new Town and Country Planning Act which did much to simplify and consolidate the real movement towards the creation of New Towns had taken place through the appointment of a Committee to advise on policy. Three reports were issued at speed, and by 1946 the New Towns Act had crystallized government policy, and thus virtually laid the foundations of the New Towns, and determined their mode of development by the Corporations set up by statute.

The financing of the Corporations was a matter for the central government, and the strict interpretation by the Minister of Housing and Local Government of Section 12(7) of the 1946 Act has tended to delay the provision of community centres and other amenities, with the result that unnecessary difficulties have been placed in the way of achieving social integration. More specifically, Section 12(7) reads:

> It shall be a condition of the making of advances to a development corporation under this section that the proposals for development submitted to the Minister under section three of this Act shall be approved by the Minister with the concurrence of the Treasury as being likely to secure for the corporation a return which is reasonable, having regard to all the circumstances, when compared with the cost of carrying out those proposals.

This is precisely where the shoe pinches: the construction of community centres, cinemas, and other amenities was sadly wanting when some of the New Towns and new estates were opened for residence. This was emphasized courageously in the Report of the Stevenage Corporation for 1953-54, in which they state that they have . . .

> Experienced much difficulty in obtaining the sanction of your Ministry for the erection of community buildings under the New Towns Act. Increasingly, in the result, has the rapidly growing population had to be content with unsatisfactory makeshifts.

* These functions are now carried out by the Ministry of Housing and Local Government.

This is destructive to that spirit of voluntary enterprise upon which the organization of communal activities so largely depends.

Surely a too rigid interpretation of this sub-section is like spoiling the ship for a hap'orth of tar, and this is one of the main causes of boredom in these areas—and idleness, and mischief.

THE TALE OF DESTRUCTION

The story of damage repeats itself in one town after another. Yet there is a difference of emphasis. The principal types of anti-social conduct observed in all kinds of housing schemes could be grouped simply as follows:

Growing things such as trees, bushes, hedges, flowers and grass verges;

buildings in the course of construction, and untenanted property;

structures in bad repair;

(less frequently) public buildings such as community centres, lavatories, telephone booths, and even schools.

There were certain interesting differences in type of damage in New Towns, compared with the estates. In the latter there was a tendency for undisciplined gangs from other parts to enter completed buildings and cause havoc. Destruction of new lifts in Liverpool flats is a bad case in point. Organized expeditions to outlying new estates also caused much injury to completed property. In the New Towns, on the other hand, the destructive impulses were directed almost exclusively to buildings under construction, or to emergency huts and sheds put up by contractors. Several reasons have been put forward to account for this difference. In the first place the provision of industries in the New Towns gives the inhabitants a common interest in the place from the start, whereas in the estates the factory is still at a distance, and many of the workers have to travel by public transport. Secondly, the New Town Corporations, in the knowledge that their clients were citizens in the full sense, consciously aimed at providing staff and services for all aspects of living. And thirdly, the age-groups represented in the New Towns consisted for the time being of a very large proportion of children under five years, a moderate number of school children, and very few adolescents. The reason for this is that the great majority of those who set out for the New Towns were young couples who had just begun to build up a family. In the New Estates, on the other hand, the families were already on entered housing lists and their age distribution was more akin to that of the ordinary population. So, for the present at any rate, the damage in the New Towns is less in extent and severity than in the estates developed by the housing authorities. The increasing number of adolescents in the New Towns may alter this balance and so create fresh problems.

Damage done by adolescents is at once more sinister and less predictable than children's pranks. As is well known, many of the most notorious of them roam about in gangs, and the harm they do is deliberate, malicious, and generally extensive. On account of the organization in gangs the depredations tend to occur in sporadic form. They show evidence of some sort of planning, however crazy they may be in execution. A great deal has been written about gang activities, and particularly good studies have been undertaken to demonstrate the essence of gang warfare. The essential characteristic of gang damage is that it is peculiarly senseless. A short time ago a hundred and fifty gravestones in the principal cemetery of Boston (Mass.) were overturned by a gang of youths, and smaller adventures in desecration have recently taken place much nearer home.

Anti-social conduct is usually annoying, but gang destruction seems as a rule to be aimed at hurting the feelings of the largest possible number of people and outraging the moral sense. Its object, in other words, seems to be to win condemnation, and the gang thrives on social disapproval. It has been said, and is probably true, that leaders of gangs make a keen study of the local press, and whenever they find that one or other of their activities has been condemned with special vehemence, they tend to repeat the offence, if possible in a more obnoxious form. Theft, although it may occur, is not the primary interest of the adolescent gang; they are much more concerned with senseless destruction. Nevertheless, as was clearly shown in a recent Glasgow study, gang raids by relatively innocent youngsters may serve as cover for professional burglars.

Many gangs glory in their work and try to become known by name. They cherish publicity and seek to engender fear. A short time ago the number of watchmen in a new town had to be trebled on account of a wave of damage by vandals. These young people painted their chosen name on the tiled floor of a new house. Timber, tools and bricks were stolen, and windows and drains were smashed. Vehicles and even cement mixers were started up at night, and barriers were erected on roadways.

In another outbreak the gangs entered houses which had been left empty during the winter months. They stole nothing, but they systematically wrecked all the furniture and fittings, smashed dishes and poured out the contents of bottles and jars, carefully avoiding actions that could be seen from the outside. It might be weeks before the damage was discovered.

Our main concern, however, is not with organized gangs but with the simpler activities of adolescent groups bent on mischief. In such instances the outbreaks of violence are more casual, depending no doubt on undesirable leadership rather than any binding organization. In new estates as well as old, for example, there are frequent outbreaks of damage to public lavatories. Probably the chief reason for this is that they are easy targets, in England at any rate. For adolescents there may well be deeper psychological associations which could be explained readily enough on Freudian principles. The amount of destruction is generally considerable: woodwork is defaced and often removed; fittings are persistently taken, and there is repeated damage to roof lights and water pipes; and toilet apparatus is smashed on the spot.

Other targets for destructive teenagers include public buildings of every kind, so long as they are left unguarded. These include clinics, community centres and clubs, municipally owned sports fields and their pavilions, and so on. One notable distinction is that damage by school children tends to be continuous and persistent, and can be anticipated and dealt with to some extent, but destruction by teenagers is sporadic and much more vicious in intensity and speed. Gang raids are usually directed to a single object, and on examination show clear signs of deliberate planning. 'This is a smash and grab raid', wrote one gang on the door of a sports pavilion which they had destroyed, although in fact nothing was taken.

The Contribution of Girls

To what extent do girls play a part in wanton destruction? We do not know, but we think that their part varies from age to age and from place to place. In the pre-school period there is nothing to choose between them. During the school years the overwhelming responsibility lies, we feel sure, with 'little wanton boys' of all social groups. As adolescence approaches, the influence of girls, at least as inciters, progressively increases, and not a few of them belong to groups of mischief makers or even organized gangs. There is much less damage in senior schools for girls than in mixed or boys' schools, and it is generally less persistent and less destructive. This is no doubt a simple demonstration of the fact that boys are more adventurous than girls; it is not of itself an indication of moral superiority.

CAUSES OF DAMAGE

Ascertainment of the causes of damage to New Towns and estates must always be a matter of opinion. We have been careful in our enquiries to take as many opinions as possible, based on the widest variety of experience. Our observations have been used to test and supplement opinion. All our informants had some direct association with these new housing developments—as tenants, members or officers of Corporations or Housing Authorities, Ministers of Religion, school teachers, medical practitioners, community wardens, probation officers, youth leaders and voluntary workers. On many matters there was complete agreement throughout, but now and again a particular interest or quality of experience brought out some unusual angle or point of view. What we are trying to disclose is not the injury itself, but 'the moving why they do it'—the immediate and the more fundamental cause of damage. First, we should like to differentiate between the personal and the environmental origins.

Personal Factors

On the personal side one of the most striking features of the enquiry has been the influence of simple boredom. This has many roots. In a great number of the areas visited a considerable proportion of the mothers went out to work, either in a factory or shop on a full-time basis or in local part-time employment. In the latter case the mother is usually able to make arrangements to return home before the children arrive from afternoon school. When whole-time employment is undertaken, arrangements are seldom made for the children to be cared for during the 'lonely' period between four and six in the evening. Only too often the mother is tired out when she reaches home at last, and is in no mood to do more than prepare a hasty meal. In some of the established areas to which new estates have been attached a long-standing tradition of women's work exists, and the young mothers are able to make arrangements for their children to be looked after by relatives, or by agreement with other women who are on shift work. In these areas, however, the number of available helpers is much greater than in the New Towns, where grannies are rare. The child is liable to suffer unless care is taken to avoid loneliness and the anti-social conduct which is apt to follow in its wake. Probably the best solution would be part-time work for the mother, but this is by no means always possible to arrange. In some cases children are actually locked out of house and home while parents are away at work, and this presents a really serious situation from the point of view of damage alone. Where there are older children arrangements are often made for one of them to have the key of the house, and this may at least prevent roaming and mischief.

A headmaster told us of one of his eight-year-old pupils who was told to go home and change to return later in the evening for a school entertainment. The little boy replied that he could not get into his home until after six o'clock when his parents returned from work. Another little boy was brought up before the Magistrates on a charge of window breaking. Until he was discovered, this form of damage had been going on for a considerable period. On enquiry it was found that the child was locked out of his home during the whole day, while his parents were at work, and they did not return until after six o'clock. It is little wonder that the boy had run wild. This period after school hours was a direct incentive for mischief.

Among adolescents the problem of boredom may be acute and its results in terms of damage are certainly extensive. In a New Town or estate the want of a community centre or even some simpler focus of interest which provides space under cover practically forces these young people into the street. Some of the New Towns have been slow in providing these important facilities for recreation indoors, and large areas have been built and occupied before any steps have been taken to meet these requirements. Unfortunately there has not been a clear-cut division of responsibility for setting up these centres, with the result that construction tends to be delayed until a harmful pattern is established. It is in this gap of time that bad habits are likely to be formed, and when a tradition of damage has once been accepted it is difficult to eradicate. The lack of social amenities such as cinema, playing fields, youth clubs, dance halls and cafes leads to the formation of idle groups among older children and adolescents.

The indications are that television is beginning to have an anomalous reaction among teenagers. At first the novelty of the apparatus brought the whole family into a long twilight of viewing, but more recently interests of the various age-groups have begun to diverge. The younger folk are becoming frankly bored with long plays, variety performances, talks and the like. The older generation still pore over the set for long periods every evening in what is probably the only sitting room, and young people rush away impatiently to take refuge in the street.

Children from good homes may also fall into habits of destruction. It has been said with a good deal of basic truth that children who have received an enlightened upbringing usually have boundless energy and daring which must be given scope. These children would be shocked at the idea of theft or any real delinquency, and yet they often show lack of social responsibility. In a city famous for its great University a considerable amount of damage was caused to trees and lawns, and the windows of many outhouses were smashed. A watch was set and it was found that the gang consisted almost entirely of the teenage sons of professors and senior lecturers in the University. Ample provision had been made for the recreational needs of the younger students, but none for the children of their teachers.

Simple questioning often leads to the answer that there is not enough for children to do in the new estates, but it is difficult to reconcile this answer with the great varieties of conduct between one estate and another, or one New Town and another, or even between the different parts of the same estate. It is often hard to know why a bad tradition springs up— whether it is due to the existence of a small group of children whose leadership is perverted, or perhaps even a single child who has talent for mischief. In some cases we were struck with the effect of adult misguidance, and in others with the apparent resentment of an old established area towards the newcomers. In the New Towns at any rate the most obvious difficulty is sheer want of community spirit.

Some new estates suffer the unfortunate experience of being singled out by the press and the public as trouble spots, and every happening receives undue publicity. Sometimes the principle of 'give a dog a bad name' begins to apply. In the New Towns this kind of selective press condemnation is not noticeable, but the towns themselves are subject to frequent criticism from the outside: 'New Towners invade old world village and destroy fences and lamp posts'. In point of fact the shoe is often on the other foot, but the old inhabitants generally escape condemnation mainly because the new has greater news value. Admittedly adverse commentary may strengthen community ties by stimulating local patriotism, but this is an unhappy way of securing positive results.

Many of the above are observations of a general character. When one comes down to the investigation of a single misdemeanour causing damage, particularly in the acts of the two younger age groups, the immediate cause is all too frequently lack of supervision by the parents. This may be due to personal factors, as we have seen, such as simple lack of attention because both parents are at work. More positive reasons include neglect, cruelty, family discord, as well as such intrinsic factors as mental deficiency, frustration or resentment in the child.

ENVIRONMENTAL FACTORS

Rubble and trouble? The physical environment has a considerable part to play in the causation of damage. Let the builder leave a heap of rubble beside a roadway and it will be pounced upon within the hour—and widely distributed. There can be little doubt that derelict areas must have had an appeal to children since time immemorial. In Britain, however, recent experiences have increased both temptation and opportunity. During the second world war vast areas of cities were partly demolished by enemy action, and children grew up in a wilderness of destruction. The bombed area was their adventure playground and it offered wonderful opportunities even for some kind of constructive play—such as building shelters or dugouts. At worst, the children, having become accustomed to violence and destruction, spent their time throwing stones and broken timber around. When the war came to an end, a great number of new estates were laid out in the neighbourhood of bombed sites, and in this way a new generation of children made their playgrounds out of demolition. The transition was quite normal when new buildings were being erected by local authorities, and so fun and games causing damage to unfinished buildings seemed quite a normal procedure. It was a simple extension of a demolition area to set about the wrecking of unfinished houses on new estates. Not only this, but many gaunt untenanted houses were helped to destruction by children from surrounding areas.

When the New Towns came to be developed, building policy led to the construction of a large number of dwellings before play spaces and other amenities had been provided. As each section of a New Town was tenanted the most obvious outlet for adventure was in the areas still under construction. Considering this it is indeed remarkable that so little damage has been recorded during the building process. The distressing feature has been the amount of damage done to growing things.

As we have seen, the risk of damage to the physical structure is increased where there are houses still under construction when tenants move into completed dwellings nearby. In the same way a housing area, which has been well prepared in advance by skilled landscaping and made attractive by the laying out of grass lands and the planting of trees and flowers, is less likely to suffer from wanton damage than an estate which is virtually a desert of wet clay and rubble for some time after occupation. We found that in a number of New Towns where no turf had been laid and where the paths and footways were ill-defined, both children ann adults ignored the restrictions which were subsequently imposed, perhaps months later, by regular planning, and failed to appreciate the artistic use of shrubberies and grass areas.

In one of the New Towns where very little damage has been recorded, it was noted that landscape planning had been completed and turf laid before the tenants moved in. In other towns the immediate surroundings of the houses have been well preserved, except where faults in planning occurred. Some New Towns report that short-cuts through shrubbery have been taken as a means to reach telephone kiosks or bus stops. Interference of this kind may be considered as natural and reasonable. The proximity of the fifth of November in England, or the twelfth of July in Northern Ireland, or of Christmas anywhere in the United Kingdom puts a considerable strain upon children who are minded to pull up hedges or shrubbery for bonfires, or fir trees for decoration. This is not a particular temptation of the New Towns alone. A more serious difficulty arises from children who have suddenly been transplanted from city life to a rural area. They have not grown up with an understanding of nature: they do not appreciate that (as Basil Spence pointed out) it takes a quarter of an hour to cut down a tree, but a quarter of a century to replace it. In some of the New Towns saplings were wantonly cut down as fencing foils or (under adult influence), as pea stakes for the garden. It takes time and education for the town child to gain a respect for growing things.

Tempting targets? In some cases the authorities placed street name plates close to the ground, and in certain suburbs the tenants imitated this arrangement in the naming of their houses. The temptation to pull out or damage signs of this kind is irresistible. Steep banks in front of houses, on which grass has been sown, are often tempting targets for damage. They form a substitute for sandpits, and children dig holes and only too easily deface the entire frontage. On sites like this, in which ground descends steeply from a roadway, some authorities have been obliged to lay the surface with pebbles.

It has been brought to our notice more than once that in buildings such as schools and clubs, fittings of poor quality are more apt to be damaged than those which are soundly constructed and fixed. In a community hall in one New Town the coat pegs in the men's cloakroom were badly attached to the wall. One peg was detached, probably inadvertently, and within a matter of days the whole lot were pulled off. It is worth noting that no damage occurred to the same fittings in the girls' cloakroom. In another town the fittings, although strongly fixed, were of poor quality. Before long one of the hooks bent under the weight of a heavy overcoat, and it was only a matter of hours before every hook was bent and twisted by the young people who used the ha'l. These are simple illustrations of the well known fact that weak fittings of poor quality do not pay, and worse still they are a positive temptation to wanton damage.

THE FOUNDATIONS OF PREVENTION

PREVENTION THROUGH INFORMAT ON SERVICES FOR ADULTS

In considering preventive measures the first and most important approach is through education, in the widest sense. The successive steps in dealing with adults are as follows: the first is to ensure that early contact is made with the new tenants before they leave their old homes. At this stage the most they are likely to know is that the industry in which the head of the family is employed has tentatively agreed to transfer its factory. The workers are consulted and a substantial number of them accept the proposals on the understanding that they will both live and work in a new town which is about to be constructed. At this point it is of great importance that representatives of the Corporation, as a housing authority, should get into personal touch with the prospective tenants. In this way the administrative officer and his staff can help to build up a positive interest in the New Town, and explain the advantages of the move. Even at this early date many questions are sure to arise in the tenant's mind, and many could be answered at the right time, and so avoid trouble and misunderstanding later on. These would apply to such diverse subjects as schools, churches, shops and their accessibility, and transport facilities.

It is always difficult to visualize information by speech or writing, so one of the first efforts in the stage of building should be to set up a properly furnished demonstration house, or preferably a series of dwelling units of differing design, and to encourage the tenants to pay personal visits to the site. This will inevitably give rise to more questions, a considerable number of which could only be effectively answered on the spot. An information office should therefore be established as soon as possible on the site, and staffed by officers who are well-versed in every aspect of New Town development. Knowledge in advance, given in a sympathetic manner, will go far to prevent subsequent misunderstanding and resentment.

When a substantial number of houses have been made ready for occupation and the tenants have moved in, they should be welcomed at the earliest possible moment by a representative of the management and so made to feel that they are already part of a living community. The feeling that someone cares means a great deal. The issue of a simple tenant's handbook during the formative period of the town's development is a good preventive measure: more elaborate editions can follow in due course. A brief pamphlet is more likely to be digested than a large, closely printed volume.

From tenant's handbooks it is a short step to Neighbourhood Newspapers, printed by the Corporation of the New Town. Some of these have a wide circulation because they are delivered free by the Corporation. They give information about the progress of the town, and its church and club activities. Many of them also serve as a vehicle for editorial propaganda about such matters as community spirit, the value of neighbourhood areas, and the importance of doing everything possible to preserve the countryside from wanton damage.

TRAINING CHILDREN IN SOCIAL RESPONSIBILITY

The first and in the long run the most important element in preventing damage by young children is the simple and gradual training in social responsibility which the parents can give in the home. There are, of course, many aspects of this training, but our interest is met by teaching little children to respect growing things and especially flowers and shrubs. One valuable method of doing this is to take advantage of the strong imitative habits of the small child. If he sees his mother, in house and garden, carefully tending flowers and other growing things, he is likely to follow her example. That is one

o

of the great advantages of having flowers in the house: the child can help to gather them intelligently and even to arrange them from a very early age. This involves a certain risk that children will learn to protect the flowers of their own garden, and at the same time be quite indifferent to other people's flowers and shrubs. One little girl began to make a habit of bringing in flowers to her mother from neighbours' gardens. This kindly activity has unfortunately to be frowned upon.

The value of parental training applies to other forms of property. Small children have to be taught to distinguish between what is their own and what belongs to other people. The use of toys is an easy and profitable object lesson as children grow out of babyhood. They can learn to respect other children's toys and this is made much easier if part of the daily play activity consists of tidying up and putting away their own toys. This raises a point that it is worthwhile all through childhood that each child should have a place of his own, even if it is only a box or a corner of a cupboard.

Children vary in their habits of tidiness and one must not be too strict about this. A sharp distinction must be drawn between simple untidiness and actual destructive habits. The destructive tendencies are probably natural enough and may well begin with a child's own toys or property. If this is left unchecked it may well spread to other children's toys and even to the family furniture. There is a point at which the parents' authority must intervene in spite of all that is said today about giving free scope to children's play.

The same is true of nursery and infant schools. A comment by Aldous Huxley is to the point: 'Modern schools may be too 'modern' by half. There is a danger that children may be given more freedom than they can profitably deal with, more responsibility than they desire or know how to take. To give children too much freedom or responsibility is to impose a strain which many of them find distressing or even exhausting'.* There is a story of a little girl who was sent to one of the very modern schools. In the course of time the mother visited the school. The child seemed unhappy, and soon gave way to tears: 'Oh Mummy,' she sobbed, 'I only wish things would be *ordinary.*'

* Huxley, Aldous: *Ends and Means.*

Training Prospective Parents

How and where can parents be trained? The ideal time, we think, is on the threshold of adolescence. At that time both boys and girls can be taught and are interested in housecraft. In some schools one or two cottages have actually been purchased for this purpose. In them the senior girls are taught routine household duties, including bed-making, cleaning, preparation and service of meals on a family scale, using the ordinary equipment of a small house. Through the cottage and its services they can also be taught laundry work and the general care of infants and young children. The cottages are also used for boys of the same age group. They are taught to handle household equipment and to do small repairs. They learn, for example, of the uses and dangers of electric and gas apparatus, and about simple household tasks. In this way both boys and girls, at an extremely impressionable age, learn the art of running a home. All this helps these young people to appreciate the importance of good maintenance, especially of property which does not belong to them.

The Young Mother

We have expressed the view that the ideal period for training prospective parents is in early adolescence. Nevertheless we should not neglect the opportunity of guidance, especially of the mother with her first child. During pregnancy and the first months of infant care these young mothers are generally in a very receptive frame of mind, and teaching through the medium of the ante-natal and infant welfare clinics can be a most valuable experience. The family doctor, a nurse, and voluntary workers can often play a considerable part in teaching infant care. A good beginning gives a young mother confidence which sustains her through many a crisis.

Group Teaching

Some form of co-operative or community care of children has become imperative which will bring children together so that they learn to carry on play and other activities as a group. This is best carried out under the influence of a nursery school in which understanding of a child's needs and the provision of outlets for his activities, constructive or destructive, is made with skill and purpose. Here we should remember Plato's caution: 'Do not use compulsion, but let early education be a sort of amusement; you will then be better able to find out the child's natural bent'.*

The reputed disadvantages of nursery schools are:

1. They take off the shoulders of the parents a burden of teaching and training.

2. They bring children together in such a way as to destroy the special influence of the home and family—i.e. by sacrificing the family to the group.

3. They increase the risks of spreading infectious diseases.

As regards the first point it is a matter of everyday knowledge that the majority of parents are not skilled to undertake this burden, and it would be better in the interests of the child to offer skilled training. It may be said that home care provides a special quality of affection which cannot be reproduced in a nursery school, but the plain fact is that a large number of mothers go out to work and could not provide the desirable care and affection in any case. The affection which they are able to provide could therefore be lavished only in the morning and evening and at week-ends—when the children are not in nursery schools. For the working mother this combination of personal home care with safe and intelligent nursery school facilities seems ideal.

On the second point there is a great deal to be said in favour of the concept of family life in which father and mother and children are all joined together, but this is feasible today only for limited periods. The nursery school is of the utmost value in training small children to live and play in groups, for this form of co-operation cannot be learned too soon after the second birthday.

The third point is hardly relevant to our study, but it does appear to us that group training in habits of cleanliness and the institution of regular orderly meals has a practical value which probably outweighs the rather theoretical risks of infectious diseases. In the modern nursery schools the children are kept in small groups. There is no assembly.

The transition from simple group instruction through play in nursery schools to school teaching proper should be a gradual

* Plato: *Republic*, Book VII.

and hardly noticeable process. Children who have already had the benefit of group training are readily distinguishable from those who have come straight from isolated homes and from playing in the streets, if only because they show far more companionship and tendency to play together. It has been said that the first difficulty of the infant school teacher is to fit children into any kind of community when their play during the previous two or three years has been so casual and purposeless.

POSITIVE PREVENTIVE TEACHING

In the right setting a great deal of preventive work can be done in the schools themselves. One good approach to this in the New Towns is through the creation of loyalties to the school itself. One headmaster of a large new school informed us that in his view it was very important to achieve this sense of loyalty to the school as a whole before attempting to create any sub-divisions (e.g. school houses). The latter carried the risk of putting rivalry in front of loyalty.

Direct instruction aimed at the prevention of damage is probably not very effective in this age group. A much better approach has been secured through encouraging a positive interest in country pursuits and nature. One of the New Towns has issued an excellent little book called 'Country Code', written in simple form so that even the youngest child can understand the story told by the pictures. But it is meant for all children of school age. The simple drawings carry a very clear message: for example, one demonstrated a child pulling down a sapling by attempting to climb it. The caption says 'Trees are to enjoy, not to destroy'. There are also straightforward warnings about fire danger and some useful hints about trees: 'Trees are alive like people. If their branches are broken or their bark cut they will die. Full grown trees are so big you can walk underneath them without hurting them, but when very young they are so small and tender—only a few inches high— that if you run about amongst them you will step on them and kill them'.

Apart from the activities of the Corporation, schools themselves can give a great deal of practical help. The children of this age group can be taught to take a great interest in growing things by helping in school gardens or by keeping gardens themselves on the school premises. Similar results can be obtained by simple competitions in bulb growing, and children are often encouraged to bring flowers of their own gathering to decorate the classroom. In this way an appreciation of wild flowers through gathering them and identifying them year by year creates a continuing interest in growing things. Further afield, many school teachers are arranging for children to be taken on expeditions to woods and forests, famous gardens and nurseries, so they learn to see each stage in planting, growth and development. One headmaster maintained interest in trees throughout the year by taking photographs of them at each succeeding season, and so taught the children to identify trees in every stage of their cycle. Another headmaster, greatly upset by wanton damage done by his pupils, put up on his school walls vivid pictures—before and after—of trees and shrubberies, grass verges and flower beds which had suffered careless injury. These pictures, which were regularly changed, served to increase the awareness of harm done.

On the positive side of prevention a great deal has been done with imagination and success. In one New Town the building of the school was not complete when the children had to move in, much of the school area was therefore out of bounds, but the imaginative headmaster met the risk of damage halfway by taking the children round the school at regular intervals so that they could see the building in progress. He kept them informed of the developments by addressing them at morning assembly and giving them an account of the work as it proceeded. In addition, when the floor of the new hall was being laid, he arranged for groups of children to see the actual construction, and when the hall was finally opened, representatives of the builders were present at the dedication service. This had been a clear temptation to damage. The headmaster, by interesting the children in the constructive work, transformed the temptation into enthusiastic co-operation.

In another of the New Towns the Chief Estates Officer, who takes a great personal interest in preserving woods and open spaces, took positive action in relation to the original village school, the frontage of which was laid with asphalt. He approached the local council with a plan for improving the school grounds with flower beds and trees and was told that it would be a waste of time. The children would destroy the young growth in a week. However, he struck a bargain with the Council that the Development Corporation would dig and prepare the area if the Council would make itself responsible for planting trees and flowers and maintaining them. Securing the co-operation of the teachers, he talked to each class and told them that if they preserved the new flower beds and grass area, they would remain as a permanent heritage. The children evidently kept their part of the bargain and the trees and flower beds are now well established.

Teaching and Practice

Some of these methods may be severely practical and the appeal to nature is by no means the only approach to damage prevention. In one school a teacher ingeniously introduced simple arithmetical sums illustrating in real terms the cost of replacing a tree or replanting a flower bed by taking into consideration the original value and the loss of time in unfruitful growth. By this means the children were made aware of the loss in terms of money value, and it might well be that a more vivid lesson was brought home to the parents than by any talk of natural beauty.

Substitutes for Prohibition

The prevention value of strict discipline in schools is questionable. The threat of the cane may deter many of the less adventurous, but it is not likely to affect the bold—especially if it is seldom carried into effect. Similarly, lectures condemning wanton damage are not likely to go very deep, and may indeed stimulate action in the opposite direction. An excess of rules is self-defeating. This matter may safely be left over until we discuss the remedial value of punishment. Of course, one of the best outlets for superabundance of energy is organized play such as football and cricket, basket-ball and hockey. Athletic sports outside and a good gymnasium indoors are no less valuable.

Planting Trees for Time to Come

'Ye shall come into the land and shall have planted all manner of trees.' Tree planting ceremonies have been introduced from time to time as a method of protection, in the hope that people will take an interest in them and hold them in respect. The results have been disappointing. On one new estate which we saw a carefully chosen public space was laid out with trees to celebrate the Coronation. Plaques were placed beneath each one to commemorate the occasion. Now, in spite of attempts at replacement, the plaques are the only memorials, giving it all the appearance of a graveyard. Similar disasters on a smaller scale have been shown to us in some of the New Towns. The adoption of trees by individuals has also proved disappointing, as this method has given rise to rivalries in which the tree itself was the principal victim. The chief hope for success lies in continuity of interest: children not only take part in planting the trees but are also responsible for maintenance. A number of teachers have formed 'associations' of children for the specific purpose of securing continued care and preservation of woods and forests.

The Value of Playspaces

There are a number of practical alternative measures to combat damage in the New Towns. So far as play-spaces are in issue there are two points of view. On the one hand it is said that there are too many open spaces in some New Towns which do not serve any useful purpose. They add to the time and effort of the tenants in getting to the shops or the post office, while they do little to attract children as real playgrounds. Most of them are not intended as play-spaces and they are not suitable in any case. It is only because they are near the homes that they attract the children at all. They should be allowed to remain undisturbed as part of the landscape planning.

The other school of thought *intend* the children to have these spaces as a playground, using the same line of argument as J. B. Russell put forward seventy years ago: 'My warning is that you working men should remember that for you the most useful open spaces are those which are close to your dwellings. Observe I do not object to those distant parks in themselves, but solely as substitutes for the occasional simple playground in the heart of the city. Both together form a complete provision for your young children whenever they can venture out during a sunny hour, as well as for yourselves on Saturday afternoons and holidays when you can go to the park with your families. I fear corporations have hitherto as a rule spent all their rates for open spaces upon these parks, and have chiefly benefitted suburban communities of wealthy people who have congregated around them beyond the area of taxation. I praise and commend for imitation by other cities the wisdom of the Corporation of Edinburgh in not only providing parks, but also clearing and paving small areas here and there in the dense portions of the city. There your youngest children can sprawl about in the sunshine, and your older ones enjoy their games. See to it also that even in the distant pleasure grounds the flower beds do not usurp all the space, but that vacant areas are left for cricket and football. There your lads, who cannot afford to lease fields like the golden youth of the wealthy, will have the same scope for wholesome recreation. Parks should not be places for merely dawdling along looking at flowers or admiring grass through iron railings.'[4]

REMEDIAL AND DETERRENT MEASURES

POLICE SUPERVISION

The sight of the policeman is undoubtedly a deterrent to the majority of youths. In the New Towns, however, there has been a delay in keeping up the police strength in proportion to the increase in population. In one new estate where the adolescents were doing much damage to public property the dearth of policemen was given as one of the reasons for it. 'When the police station was built in the area and more policemen arrived, the amount of damage decreased very noticeably', one inhabitant reports.

As regards police action a caution delivered on the spot is generally effective with the younger children; even the adolescent behaves when there is a policeman at his elbow. A simple caution from a policeman in uniform is very often all that is required in sporadic outbreaks of destruction, but a visit to the home may be even better when young children are involved. Court action is properly reserved as a rule for cases involving personal injury or really serious damage requiring compensation, or possibly leading to fine or imprisonment.

In one area with which we are familiar an attempt was made owing to the shortage of policemen to provide houses for them at strategic points in the town so that they could exercise their influence outside their hours of duty. This imposed an unfair burden on the police, and never really came into operation.

GENERAL SUPERVISION

Firm but kindly supervision is an essential feature of prevention. It is also the best deterrent, when a wave of destruction has already broken, and others are likely to follow. In one New Town the employment of two retired policemen as park keepers had an excellent effect, because they knew many of the children in the area and were held in high respect. In another area near London persistent destruction in the parks was brought to an end by the engagement of a retired physical training instructor from the Navy. In addition to his supervisory work he took a great personal interest in the boys, and taught them physical exercise. He won affection by becoming a play-leader rather than a watch-dog.

In recent years there has been an increasing tendency to appoint trained play-leaders especially for the supervision of playgrounds in which suitable apparatus has been provided. This has several advantages. It enables the leader to supervise the apparatus and to take part in maintaining the playground and perhaps the adjacent open spaces belonging to the authority, and at the same time he gets to know the children individually and thereby exercises a personal influence over their activities.

One of the difficulties in the maintenance of a *small* playground is the cost of supervision. They are often not large enough to justify the appointment of a caretaker on a full-time basis. In one city which we visited this difficulty had been met by providing, in the same area, a garden for the elderly people, three tennis courts for adults and a small children's playground close to a built-up area. This arrangement permitted full time supervision by a paid caretaker who was also able to keep an eye on the other parts of the ground. But let it be emphasized that supervision of children is not a task for the amateur, however socially minded. It calls for training and ability of a special kind.

The 'Law of Diminishing Damage,

In a number of the New Towns, when damage to young trees has occurred, it has been customary to restore the loss without making any fuss about it. The principle on which this action is founded is well described as 'the law of diminishing damage'. The theory is that much of the early destruction in the New Towns is due to curiosity and experiment rather than malice. So, when injured trees or shrubs have been replaced, the number destroyed on the next occasion is less, and in the course of time becomes negligible. One reason brought forward for this promising state of things is sheer boredom. There is no fun in destroying trees unless the action causes a stir through public condemnation. It becomes a mug's game.

Good Maintenance

There is another aspect which is more important: good maintenance is respected by all but the few incorrigibles. Money spent on trees and flowers in abundance is money well spent. Wanton damage is directed mainly towards buildings and growing things that are already defective. It is the loose brick that will be dislodged, the mortar lying about that will be thrown at walls, and the rubble that will be used to break glass. Good maintenance takes away temptation, but certain conditions must first be observed. It is no use, for example, merely to instal charming parks and leave it at that. There must in addition be some outlet for child energy. For that reason a safety valve is interposed, such as a hard playground with a blank wall against which a ball can be thrown time without end, a practice pitch for cricket, with high nets, or even a big rough patch for letting off steam.

Co-operation of the Press

We have already referred to publicity, and two dangers have raised their heads. First, that public censure is enjoyed by gangs, and secondly, that New Towns have from time to time become a target for uninformed criticism. Apart from these risks, the Press has done a great deal to popularize the New Towns by describing the services that they render and by showing photographs of their amenities. Publicity of this kind creates a positive interest in these enterprises. Although it can hardly be used as a remedial measure, it can be useful by offering censure without sensation.

NEGATIVE MEASURES

Two other remedies for damage have been employed, but their value is open to question. The first of these could be defined as the withdrawal of existing facilities—surely a humiliating procedure for a New Town. In one instance a fine private park had been thrown open to local residents, and with the arrival of the New Town, the new tenants were also included. For a time this amenity was respected, but later the owner found it necessary to tighten the regulations, because youths were lighting fires in ancient hollow trees and actually burning hay ricks on the estate. As a result of this the facilities had to be greatly restricted and partly withdrawn. In some cases a wood has had to be closed as a public amenity because of persistent damage.

In another instance a lodge has been left on the edge of a new estate, intended for use as a community hut in due course— therein lies the failure. In no time the lead had been stolen, the walls pulled down brick by brick, until the remainder became a positive danger, and the authority, accepting defeat, was obliged to remove all that was left.

On another new estate a Sunday School Mission moved out of a farm house which had been built over twenty years ago and had been occupied temporarily by the Mission for the last few years. Within an incredibly short time after the removal, when the building was left empty, it was stripped of its lead and all its windows broken, slates were ripped off and locks and door handles were removed. It is now a danger to the public and will have to be pulled down. At the time of our visit two little boys came up to us and said rather pathetically 'that used to be our Sunday School'.

The deliberate non-replacement of damaged property is to an even greater extent a gesture of defeat. It is deplorable to see a desolation of tree stumps and it is even sadder from the human point of view to be told of a youth club and children's nursery which have been abandoned because of misuse.

In one New Town we were shown a playground where there had been a hut and various other pieces of equipment. The hut had been destroyed very soon after its erection, as had some of the less strong pieces of equipment, by an older age group, and these were apparently not being replaced. It is always the innocent who suffer, as much of the damage is done by older children. It is a pity that the loss is not made good.

TRAINING IN SOCIAL RESPONSIBILITY

There is no doubt that in many cases the parents carry a heavy responsibility for the damage actually done by their children. *The parents who do not care* form a small but hard core of the neglectful; they neglect their homes and their children, and they are generally not merely socially incompetent but positively anti-social. When all is said and done, however, the majority of the parents whose children create trouble have themselves had little chance in their own upbringing. They are ignorant, and no one takes the trouble to teach them. They are dumped into new houses with all their strangeness of fittings and equipment, and no one explains how these work. How can we expect these parents to be guides to their children on the matter of social responsibility?

In the New Towns this anomaly is being increasingly recognized, and serious attempts are being made on all sides to make the art of living together a happy experience and not a burden. All the same, there are occasions when the parents must accept responsibility for their children's misbehaviour. The first and most direct measure is to make the parents pay in cash for the harm done by their children; and in point of fact it is often a good deterrent. Wherever possible this should be done without having recourse to law. Demonstrations of actual damage, shown to groups of parents through parent-teacher associations or women's institutes, may have a useful deterrent effect, and in a similar way repeated anti-litter campaigns are best appreciated by means of organized visits to the malignant spot.

RECREATION AS A MEANS OF PREVENTION

No study of damage prevention would be complete without a discussion of the influence of play, and the best means of providing for healthy recreation. Play is the natural introduction of the child to the art of living with others, and its influence continues side by side with instruction through the whole period of childhood and adolescence. Play is just as much an expression of vital activity as work. In the course of this brief chapter it will be seen that the provision for play occupies a prominent place in our programme for the prevention of damage.

The size, the situation, and the equipment of a play area depend primarily on the age of the users. The simplicity or complexity of organization varies with the purpose of use—for games or sports, for swimming and other specially designed activities which need skilled supervision. It has been said by people of long experience that even in the more simply equipped playgrounds the children will eventually lose interest and go back to the streets unless there is a grown-up on the spot to give it life and to maintain healthy interest. Supervision is admittedly expensive, but wherever buildings and equipment are provided, it is better to spend money on a leader than to be plagued with the recurring costs of renewing wantonly damaged property.

OUTDOOR RECREATION

The needs of older children (12 to 15 years) demand the provision of large fields for a variety of purposes. In the design of New Towns and estates it is important that the school playing fields should not be sited at too great a distance unless good public transport is available. Accessibility is of great value, especially if the playing fields are to be used by young workers who have recently left school. They have no time to spare for long excursions. School playing fields vary greatly in the extent of their arrangements, but practically all of them have pitches for cricket, football and hockey. Some of the modern playing fields have tennis courts and running tracks as well as arrangements for other games and athletic exercises. Changing rooms and storage accommodation for equipment are provided, and sometimes a small pavilion for spectators in addition. Many of the larger schools make arrangements, so far as they can, for former pupils; but these are usually limited to recognized clubs.

A considerable number of the larger industrial firms lay out sports grounds for their employees, and such arrangements deserve every encouragement. The expression 'sports ground' generally refers to an enclosed area owned or leased by a public authority, an organized body such as an industrial firm, or a professional or amateur club. The sports ground is reserved for a specific activity such as cricket, football or athletics, and is not as a rule open to the general public except in their capacity as spectators. As the New Towns grow and prosper one may confidently expect that sports grounds will be laid out. Our main interest in development, however, rests with the public provision of open spaces and the prevention of their wanton misuse.

The Corporations of New Towns have set aside space to be used for more or less organized games and some of the authorities are engaged in the construction of playing fields. These are not as a rule precisely laid out, although they will no doubt have pavilions, changing rooms and stores for equipment. Pitches are often used side by side by more or less organized teams of players but not to the exclusion of the general public or the small boy with a bat and ball. Some sections of these areas, especially tennis courts and bowling greens, can usually be reserved for a limited period by any group at a small charge. In addition a growing number of these public playing fields will have an open air swimming bath for which a charge would be made. This kind of playground is essentially public property and open without reserve to the inhabitants of the area.

At this point it should be emphasized that playing fields set aside for public use should not be merely open spaces; they ought to have a focus for activities, a centre of some kind from which these activities radiate. The best way of meeting this need is to construct a pavilion or shelter at the most accessible part of the area. This building should be combined with store rooms for gardening and sports equipment and it should have adequate lavatory accommodation. As the pavilion is to be built for all comers and not solely for the members of clubs and associations it must be strongly constructed and protected if it is to survive. Many of the existing shelters and pavilions built in public parks, even where there is little or no supervision, are so flimsy as to be a positive temptation to the marauder. In public playing fields these pavilions should be as indestructible as the mind of man can devise. Even the lavatory should be able to resist all attack short of explosive charges. Cisterns can be concealed behind concrete walls and their discharge controlled by push buttons set flush with the walls. No pipes of any kind need be visible at all, and it is surely not beyond the wit of the sanitary engineer to make all other fittings resistant to damage. It costs money to do this, of course, but no more in the long run than the ever recurring expenses of repair. In one area, for example, we were informed that a single public lavatory cost the local authority two hundred pounds a year for the repair of wanton damage. There remains the problem of obstruction of drains by materials deliberately pushed down water closets. This trouble can at least be minimised by the insertion of large trap covers which make clearing a simple operation.

In finding space for unorganized amusement in the open air the New Towns have a great advantage over many other estates by reason of the selected nature of their situation. They are mostly surrounded by woods and farm lands which in some towns push their long fingers between the neighbourhoods and come quite close to the dwellings. Many of these lands and woods are in private ownership, and the benefits which they offer are confined to space and open air. Public open spaces, on the other hand, are common lands dedicated to the inhabitants as a whole and not to be hired, except perhaps for some traditional activity such as a fair. It would be a great pity if such unallocated spaces were to be lost to the community. They have special importance for older children during their school life, in offering opportunities for expeditions and nature studies as part of the school programme, as well as general activities like explorations, picnics and free play. For adolescents who have left school these lands have a real value in giving room for completely unorganized play, fun and ploys of every kind without any sense of restriction. We are confident that the provision of these public open spaces would go far to obviate the damage to adjacent farm lands and equipment. At the present time this is all too common on the borders of new housing estates.

While we are considering open spaces in general it is desirable to complete the picture by a reference to formal public parks. Doubts have been raised whether these are necessary in the New Towns, where there is already abundant open space. A propos of this, it is interesting to hear that on one new housing estate the local housing authority turned a large area which was not to be scheduled for building purposes for a considerable time into an open recreation space. A paradise for youth, one would have thought. Yet there were constant requests from the tenants to have this space transformed into an orthodox public park. There are solid advantages in creating a public park so long as it is reasonably accessible to a substantial number of the inhabitants. The layout is very important; there should be a large number of trees, flower beds, paths wide enough to take two prams, and above all plenty of reasonably comfortable seats. When a park of this type is designed, a number of quite small grass plots separated from the main parkland by pathways and perhaps low fences should be set aside for very young children and provided with a number of seats for the mothers. There is a real social value in this, for it enables mothers with young children and babies in prams to sit for a while and talk to their friends while the infants sleep and the toddlers scamper around. The public parks should also provide a sense of adventure for the younger children of school age, with paddling pools, boating ponds, and fields laid out for games. All the same, beauty should not be forgotten. The public park is intended to interest people of all ages; it is the ideal site for large and variegated flower beds, flowering trees and shrubs and the rarer varieties of growth. The disadvantages are the cost of upkeep in relation to other open spaces and the risk of damage unless there is pretty close supervision.

THE INTERNATIONAL PATTERN

The pattern of damage by children and adolescents in other countries is remarkably uniform, but the extent of the problem shows wide variations. In Australia and New Zealand, for example, the total amount of damage is trivial compared with Britain and the United States, but the same old crazy pattern stands out: 'Razor Blades used to slash Carriage Seats', and again 'Vandals spoil Festival'. The latter act was done by gangs of youths who tore up flowers and decorations, and so ruined the charm of a carefully prepared flower show in a New Zealand township. The local newspapers ask, just as they do in this country: 'Have such people no thought for others? Why can they not enjoy a day's pleasure without all this nastiness?'

In the Peoples' Republics there have also been serious outbreaks of violence: senseless violence apparently associated with alcohol in some cases, and in others with racial intolerance. A similar wave has been sweeping over some of the large cities in the United States, with grave consequences in New York City, where even the older school children have got out of hand as perpetrators of senseless crime. In all this there is one element of grace: one often hears of a pathetic, misguided faithfulness to the gang. The loyalties are there, if only they could be redirected into socially acceptable channels. In many countries there is a blurred distinction between public and private property, and less sense of responsibility is shown towards what is owned by that vague body called the Authority. 'Voler l'Etat n'est pas voler' the saying goes.

In October 1955 Sweden abolished its liquor rationing system. After one year the street authorities reported that the parks of the capital had become haunts of drunken and anti-social persons to a much greater extent than ever before. One of the unfortunate sequels to this change was that proposals had to be made for fencing the public parks, as in London, Paris, Copenhagen and Moscow, and to close them at night.

It is stated that one of the characteristics of the Northern countries is that a great deal of the destruction is purposeless. On the way to the Mediterranean a subtle change occurs: 'Il est possible qu'il existe une différence entre les enfants et les adolescents des pays du Nord et d'eux des pays méditerranéens. Le comportement sauvage des gangs de jeunes aux Etats-Unis ou en Suède est incompréhensible dans un pays latin et infiniment peu probable. Ce n'est pas qu'il y ait moins de pervers et de petits débiles mentaux, mais leurs activités sont plûtot dirigées vers le vol astucieux—vers ce que les italiens appellent 'la bella combinazoine' et non vers la 'wanton destruction'.

Most of the superficial damage in towns is carried out by children from the estates themselves, but the more serious outbreaks of violence and major destruction are the work of gangs from outside. In all countries the targets are similar: telephone booths, buildings under construction, benches in parks and seats in railway waiting rooms. Cinema seats and railway carriages seem to be especially vulnerable because they are easy game and give rise to notoriety and press criticism. In most of the reports received it has been pointed out that newspaper publicity and adverse criticism is eagerly sought. This fact involves no criticism of the Press, as in the long run it is publicity that draws the people's attention to ill-doing.

The 'age-group' of damage varies little from country to country. Two periods are marked out: the school group from 8-12 years, and the juveniles of 15-21. In the earlier group most of the harm is due to the indifference of the parents, or the effects of broken homes, family quarrels, and general unhappiness in the household. In the older group the reasons are more complex. Of an African city it was said: 'There is little home life for adolescents. That is the main reason for hooliganism'. 'Blame boredom', said a Rhodesian paper, 'The boys and girls just do not have anything to do'. Want of something to do is the principal alleged cause of vandalism, but it is not the only one. In one country the reasons are set out in some detail:

> Everyone agrees that the unsettlement of social life by movement to new housing estates has a lot to do with vandalism, as with other symptoms of maladjustment. But full employment, good wages, absence of slums, plenty of space in the form of private gardens, parks, recreation grounds, beaches, mountain and bush, and a certain freedom from restrictions of any kind— all these factors probably play some part in prevention.

From another country a correspondent with long teaching experience tells us that in his view a good deal of the vandalism and other delinquent behaviour in new housing estates is only symptomatic of the difficulties with which children are faced. In a new housing area families have been recently uprooted and are thrown into a fresh environment where they have to remake all their social contacts. Such occasions are disturbing even to adults, whose tensions build up until such time as fresh social contacts are made, and the family finds its feet in the new environment. These tensions are communicated to the children, who are not only affected by them but are also facing their own difficulties in establishing *their* social contacts. The disturbance of the children leads to many forms of socially delinquent behaviour, most of which is symptomatic.

Another element in causation of damage is a large gap between school leaving age and regular employment. The disruption caused by a period of military service is apt to have a similar effect. It has always been recognized that irregular employment of young boys has a deleterious effect on their habits and outlook.

On the question of prevention there is a good deal of agreement between one country and another. Perhaps the most widespread approval is given to the two theories: that unguarded property should be strongly built to resist interference, and that damaged property ought to be replaced at once. Differing views are held on the value of preventive teaching in schools and other educational institutions. On the one hand it is urged that a great deal of educative work can be effectively carried out by co-operation between home and school. 'Youngsters *can* be taught by school, radio and television to respect public property.' Another authority in Switzerland, makes a strong plea for appropriate areas for play and exercise among school children, and above all, for those who have recently left school, otherwise the excessive vitality of these young people, who are everywhere staying 'outside' then easily takes a negative turn. The first remedy for this is to create sufficient and appropriate occupation possibilities for both these stages of life. A third report takes a more gloomy view: 'A number of attempts have been made by competent teachers to develop collective education: results negative'.

A greater diversity of opinion occurs in the assessment of remedies for wanton damage and juvenile delinquency in general. In Bulgaria it has been decided that extreme provocation demands severe measures. A wave of hooliganism culminated in an incident that shocked the people. Two young workers were on their way home in a tram, when suddenly, and without any obvious reason, one of them was attacked and stabbed fatally by two young thugs. What was so disturbing was that not one of the tram passengers showed any interest in the act and the perpetrators were allowed to go home undisturbed. Nor did any of the passengers report the incident. This gives some indication of the extent to which hooligan gangs can terrorise a neighbourhood. As a direct consequence of this crisis, a Law for combating juvenile delinquency has been introduced (18 February, 1958) and adopted by the National Assembly. A Central Commission is being set up in the Chief Prosecutor's office, with representatives of education, health and welfare. One of the functions of the Commission is to study the causes of juvenile anti-social activities, and to work out measures for re-education. The legal provisions include special schools for children above seven years, and compulsory labour schools for adolescents. Very strict measures are being taken against persons who sell alcohol to defectives or to children, and the law is being more effectively applied to deal with offences.

An investigation of the trials against hooliganism in 1956 in Sofia showed that 90 per cent of the cases were associated with the consumption of alcohol. Similar findings have been published in other Soviet countries, and the problem has reached alarming proportions in Poland, and in a number of other countries, widely scattered over the world. Nevertheless, it cannot be assumed, on the evidence available, that a successful campaign against drunkenness, desirable as it is in itself, will solve the whole question of wanton damage by children or teenage gangs. The experience of the United Kingdom and a number of other European countries denies this, and the complex situation in the great cities of the United States offers no reason for complacency, even in the absence of drink or drugs. The gangs of mere children who have been terrorizing schools in parts of New York, or behaving dangerously on suburban trains in Chicago, are not actuated by artificial stimulants, but rather intoxicated by a passion for power and notoriety. For that very reason they are offering a serious challenge to society—one which ought to be met here and now. The evidence which we have accumulated from many lands through the cordial co-operation of colleagues points unmistakeably to two conclusions which are not in conflict, yet they must not be considered separately.

The position amounts to this: During the past twelve years or so there has been (with conspicuous exceptions) a marked increase in negligent and wanton damage to property by children and in deliberate acts threatening public order and security, mainly by adolescents. Hooliganism is no doubt as old as the history of man, and it has passed through many phases of severity as a public menace in various civilizations. But today there is a new and disturbing element. It has its positive side, represented in the Press by success stories about teenage tycoons and in real life by cheerful adventure. Unfortunately the negative aspect is more prominent, for the reasons we have tried to bring together. It is unnecessary to summarize these at this stage, but perhaps the most striking feature is the power of money and the impetus it gives to young people to shake themselves free from guidance of any kind. There are faults on the side of those who criticize: impatience and want of understanding, and at the same time what de Tocqueville described with an uncanny prophetic insight as 'a kind of virtuous materialism . . . which would not corrupt but enervate the soul, and noiselessly unbend its spring of action'.[5]

The long-term attack on the position surely depends on conscious and well-directed educational measures: the nursery school, concentration in school teaching on positive interests in the natural and social sciences, and above all, a continuing endeavour to influence the growing child through good home care. But that is not enough to meet the immediate threat to the welfare of those who are on the threshold of adolescence today. There must be a short term policy depending on the better direction of leisure activities—a new outlook on education through play which works through, and not against, the changing interests of boys and girls as they enter the bewildering realm of adolescence.

GENERAL OBSERVATIONS

THE BEGINNINGS OF COMMUNITY LIFE

The distinguishing feature of the New Towns is that work is provided for the inhabitants locally. Home and work are in the same area. The consequence of this is that the families move from their own homes with a certain eagerness of anticipation, however much they regret the severing of old associations.

On *a priori* grounds there should be every reason to expect that the tenants would quickly take a pride in their new homes and settle down to the new work. This was to some extent true of the early inhabitants who felt the spirit of adventure, perhaps even with a faint hostility towards the 'natives'. Unfortunately that early feeling of common interest became overwhelmed by weight of numbers. The intimacy which had no deep roots has disappeared, and the attempts to create community life have turned out to be a hard struggle.

THE NEED FOR PROVISION IN ADVANCE

One of the most important reasons which has been brought home to us again and again is that community facilities have been just too late. The needs of the tenants are not static during the development. At first, when there is a sense of bewilderment, these needs are great and urgent, and it is just then that the time-lag has occurred. Small-scale premises would have been perfectly appropriate at that time, because they would have served a variety of interests. People really only wanted to compare notes and to discuss common problems with others; and it was no doubt wise to delay permanent building until community interests were crystallized. In the meantime, however, a beginning should have been made in a small way with the sites selected for public buildings and local play spaces. A community centre should be small to begin with, but with room for expansion. What is more, there should be plenty of them from the very start, as well as a goodly number of informal meeting points like pubs and cafes, milk bars and fish-and-chip shops. The essential principle is to provide for recreation and amenity near the people's homes; these provisions should be ready to welcome the tenants when they first arrive. The amenities should be more varied than will be ultimately required, so as to give people a sense of choice; and community centres should never be ponderously large at the start.

HINDRANCES TO COMMUNITY DEVELOPMENT

The want of provision of these amenities at the start is probably the greatest hindrance to community development, but there are other factors. As a rule there is a great deal of over-time in the factories, with the result that the workers are tired before the long day is over. This applies particularly when women go out to a full day's work, as well as their husbands. It has been suggested that the attraction of television keeps families at home and limits their outside activities. Most of our informants, such as Health Visitors and other workers who are regularly in and out of the homes of the people, believe that the strongest factor of all is that in most homes the children are too young to be left in the evening. 'Sitters-in' would no doubt be unobtainable in any number, but in point of fact they are not encouraged. In one of the New Towns a brave attempt was made to run a roster of baby sitters arranged by a voluntary agency. It did not work for several reasons. The parents did not like the idea of leaving their children in the care of 'strangers', even though the strangers lived only a few doors away. In addition, they were not taken with the idea of these strangers inspecting house and furniture and perhaps making adverse comments.

The distance and formality of the big community centres discourages early friendships. We believe strongly that more small centres and other amenities close to the homes would create a much happier atmosphere and encourage mutual help. In other words, there is a very strong case for stimulating the New Towns to make these advance provisions, and they should not be stinted in money to provide them. As one writer expressed it: 'All our experience of urban development teaches that if a town is starved of amenities in its early years, it bears the marks of that malnutrition all its life'.[6]

VARIED AMENITIES

We have referred first to community centres because they represent a recognised provision in the New Towns. At the same time we are most anxious to stress the importance of less formal and equally vital amenities. The city areas from which many of the tenants come are no doubt over-provided with shops. In the New Towns the policy is to have the main shopping centre for the town as a whole, with secondary neighbourhood groups as required by the building programme. It is uncommon to find a little shop near a group of houses where a general dealer conducts his friendly trade. Indeed, the building of these little shops is frowned upon by architects and planners on the one hand and big chain stores on the other. The reasons given for rejecting the corner shop are not very convincing. It is said, for example, that the shopkeeper cannot rely on enough custom to enable him to pay his way, but the experience indicates that authorities which have permitted general stores find that the tenants do make a good living from them, and pay an economic rent. Again, it is alleged that the general dealer would take away a substantial amount of trade from shopkeepers at the neighbourhood centres. No doubt there is some force in this argument, but in our view the balance tilts heavily on the side of the dealer. People moving to the New Towns have been accustomed to doing some of their daily shopping near at hand. One report after another tells us that this is the one amenity which is most greatly missed by the newcomer. We do believe that these little shops within easy reach of houses have a most valuable function in helping the new tenants to feel more at home. They fulfil a real social need by helping busy mothers to get goods near at hand instead of having to trail laboriously with their infants to distant shopping centres.

The nearby store allows mothers to send quite small children on shopping errands to a friendly and understanding shopkeeper, with the added comfort that they are free from traffic risks. There is a further point, not to be ignored: the little shop is a focus of interest in a street, and it has a real social value as a place for conversation—and no doubt gossip—among neighbours. In a recent report[7] a sub-committee summed up the situation as follows:

> Such shops can be satisfactorily designed as part of a corner site on a housing estate; in this position they may form a useful screen for back gardens and avoid other difficulties in the layout of corners. They might equally well form part of a block of flats, which is a common practice on the continent. Shops of this kind not only have the social and other advantages we have mentioned, but they provide a means of livelihood for some at least of the small shopkeepers displaced by slum clearance. They might serve a similar useful purpose in the case of disabled persons. We recommend local authorities to consider very carefully the more extensive provision of shops of this kind.

In the planning of New Towns we think that the case is even

stronger, because we are dealing with families with a large number of young children. The mothers lack the usual city sources of help in shopping and similar errands.

ENTERTAINMENTS

In the register of amenities we should remember the importance of pubs and cafes, as meeting places in addition to their functions of nourishing body and mind. The kindly hearts of inn-keepers induce them to encourage conversation and friendly meetings, and cafes and dance halls are moving in their fashion towards the same beneficent end. The best barriers against mischief are, first, to have something to do, and secondly, to have somewhere to go for the purpose. The cinema and the television set have their part to play in reducing the flow of anti-social conduct. There are admittedly certain reservations. Horseplay and seat-slashing has occurred in cinemas, and only too often the quality of the films shown is deplorable, especially when they make a parade of the worst side of human conduct. The quality of television programmes is frequently poor enough in all conscience, but they can hardly be accused of inciting to breaches of the peace. TV has its good points: it helps to keep the family together; it extends our knowledge and experience; it is often a useful recipe for idleness; and at its best it gives mental relief and relaxation. In a sense TV is anti-social and the question has frequently been raised of late as to whether it is not too effective in diminishing social contacts outside the home. On the other hand there are signs that the initial attraction is wearing off, especially among adolescents. Young children are still inclined to addiction. A more serious feature of the situation is that in small houses adolescents are positively driven out, because the only public room is being used endlessly for programmes that please either their parents or the younger members of the family.

LITTER

Children have an inexorable habit of throwing paper and other garbage about if it is not kept in proper containers. In one New Town an old tradition of the area has been continued and the tenants will not buy proper dustbins. Instead, they stuff their rubbish into old cardboard boxes for the collectors to take away, during which process much of it is blown all over the street. We have also seen the unfortunate results of the delivery on the roadside of commodities such as fuel, sand and bricks. Naturally these attract children, who often create a mess which takes months to clear up. We feel that the Authority should, in these instances, take stronger measures to enforce the use of proper receptacles and the quick storage of other materials. One unchecked source of damage provokes another.

MERITS OF WORK NEAR THE HOME

The New Towns are fortunate, as we have seen, in combining work and home. In this they compare very favourably with the pseudopodia of established cities where the daily travel to work has an unsettling effect, and where there is the additional anxiety among women with small children of finding a new job. If the housewife takes the alternative of giving up work altogether, the boredom itself is unsettling and reflects on her whole outlook. In the New Towns, on the other hand, the housewife has usually a reasonable choice. She may decide to devote her whole attention to home and children or to look for work. This is often readily available at no great distance from the home; and when both parents have the opportunity for work in the area it should be easier for them to settle down and take part in the making of the community.

These are theoretical considerations. The facts which we possess indicate that the evidence is rather shaky and we feel that further research is necessary to establish genuine conclusions.

CAUSES OF UNSETTLEMENT

On a large estate recently studied in which the community was economically reasonably well placed, and where there was no difficulty in securing work quite close to the new area, there were nevertheless marked signs of instability for a period of years. This was shown for example by a high initial incidence rate in juvenile delinquency, and a subsequent decline over five years to half the figure in the first year. In each year there was a progressive decline, but the significant point is that the figure came down only to the level that prevailed in the cities from which the rehoused families came. In the early years it was a good deal higher than that of the cities, so that one can conclude that large-scale rehousing produces a short phase of social dislocation, followed by recovery. Further studies are needed to show whether this goes on to positive improvement.

In the New Towns also there is definite evidence of social dislocation in the early phases of residence. Many of the tenants attribute this, probably correctly, to lack of amenities, and in some instances even of 'essential' services. The excess of damage done by children and adolescents in these early days may well be related to the same fundamental causes—the unsettling effects of the new surroundings, the lack of 'belonging', sheer curiosity about unfamiliar things, and, above all, the patent lack of play-space.

MEDICAL CARE

Among the provisions which help to bring people together in a strange town or neighbourhood is the common misfortune of sickness. Some of the New Towns have been bold in experiment; not content with a policy of drift they have secured, with voluntary help, the establishment of a health centre of the most modern type, designed to bring together under the general practitioners working as a group, the care of family health. This is an exciting advance on the older concepts of employing a doctor to attend upon individual sickness. The combination of infant and school health centres with general family care is one of the marks of the new society.

SETTLING DOWN

The process of settling down is a very delicate one. At the time of the move there is, of course, a great deal of pleasurable excitement, mingled with a none too happy anticipation of change and the loss of familiar people and surroundings. For several months at least there is a thrill associated with the new home and its furnishings. A different way of living has to be learnt, and the younger couples usually enjoy it. But for a long time they do not look on the town, or even the house, as their own. It is as though they had come on a prolonged visit, and they still think and act as if the old, busy city were their real dwelling-place. In the early days of the Corby development the workers, who came mainly from Motherwell, had no great feeling of loyalty to their new town for some time. On every holiday there was no discussion as to where the period should be spent. It was Motherwell as a matter of course. As the years wore on, however, and the older generation at home began to die out, a conflict arose between Scotland and the Lincolnshire coast. It is believed that the change of outlook took some eight to ten years to complete.

There are other personal factors which tend to draw the people towards their new home. Gradually many of them begin to take a genuine pride in the garden—and it is just at that time they begin to complain of the want of fences or hedges around their fronts. Then there is the strong urge to keep up with the Jones family, a motive that brings curtains to the windows and polish to the front doorstep. This keeps them busy for some time, but it does not encourage them to take any part in community life. We keep ourselves to ourselves. So, in the course of time the women, who have no attachment to any place of work, feel keenly the lack of friends. Even those who do go out to work have difficulty at this stage in forming associations with their neighbourhood and home environment. In their fascinating book 'Family and Kinship in East London' the authors quote the following interview:

> . . . the husband was congratulating himself on having a house, a garden, a bathroom, and a TV—'the telly is a bit of a friend down here'—when his wife broke in to say—'It's all right for you. What about all the time I have to spend here on my own?'[8]

We do not know how long it takes to settle in a New Town. The subject deserves further study. It is clear that the children make friends far sooner than their parents, no doubt mainly because their roots in the old home are not nearly so deep; but the fact that they go to play and school together makes for easy intimacy. As a rule there are few neighbourhood difficulties, as children are not so choosy. The street and the nearby play-space are friend-makers. This adds something to the speed of settling, but more is needed. It takes a longer time for the children to feel that the neighbourhood is their own, and not the property of some indifferent stranger. That is one of the reasons why the children, chiefly through curiosity and a passion for exploring, do a lot of damage in the early months, damage which they would not dream of doing in their homes. For some time the new neighbourhood seems a fair target, and city children are slow to recognize that growing things are set for their enjoyment, and not as objects for destruction.

HELP FROM THE AUTHORITIES

In the process of settling down, the two major authorities— that is, the Development Corporation and the Local Authority —can do much to facilitate the movement. We have already indicated that in our view there should be both a large community centre for the town as a whole, and a number of small units for neighbourhood use, but how much ought to be laid on by the authority and how much provided through the initiative of the people themselves? This is really fundamental, because it determines a very crucial point. Are the inhabitants going to talk eternally about 'They' and never about 'we'? We have noticed again and again that tenants' associations tend to be grumbling associations, and their pressure groups attempt to force 'Them' (that is the authority) 'to do something about it' instead of trying to solve the difficulty through their own group action. In other words, they have not yet identified themselves with the life of the town. If this process goes on indefinitely it makes for unrest, and even indifference to the actual destruction of property which 'They' ought to replace, according to tenant opinion.

How can we best transform 'Them' into 'us'? The authority must provide the fundamentals such as playing space and accommodation, but it is unreasonable and wrong in practice, to expect them to be responsible for organizing the various activities to be carried on. One of the least excusable of all cries is: 'They don't provide anything for us to do'. It is only fair to say, however, that tenants' associations, as soon as they understand the real position, begin to foster the community spirit and to encourage initiative in clubs and other recreational activities. In this advance to social co-operation they are helped by a wealth of voluntary societies. For some years, unfortunately, the keen voluntary workers are few in numbers, and their names appear on a whole series of committees. Gradually the new families will be brought in, although at first they are so engrossed in home and family that they can hardly be persuaded to join in anything.

THE PLACE OF VOLUNTARY ASSOCIATIONS

In the development of voluntary organizations the Corporations have been most helpful. Without the active encouragement of their staff (and wives) it would hardly have been possible to breach the formidable wall of isolation. The residents of a New Town are very dependent on their own voluntary efforts for recreation and help in time of trouble, but at first they hesitate on the brink. It is just at this point that the Corporations have provided the essential stimulus. The New Towns are in fact a fine test of the capacity for community planning. It is not easy to get going because the newcomers have so many distractions—in setting up a home and a garden and in providing for the care of young children. In spite of this they have done well and one need not be anxious about the very large number of associations. Trial and error is the best method where there is abundant energy and enthusiasm. Apart from the shop and the factory, voluntary associations are the best means of creating new friendships, and many of them are valuable in bringing the children together out of school hours, and free from the necessary discipline of education.

In matters of this kind the Corporations have gladly accepted the function of maintaining close contact with the tenants, at least in their early years. They have taken the trouble to listen patiently to complaints and even when they have not been able to put things right they have explained the difficulties in such a way as to satisfy all but the most outrageous tenants. In addition they have accepted responsibility for many practical things such as landscaping, care of the open gardens, and assistance for town dwellers in the unusual task of making a back garden.

It may be argued that paternalism on the part of the Corporations has been carried too far, and that too much assistance, for example, has been given to the creation and running of voluntary associations. Some of the New Towns have several hundred of them. It has even been suggested that the amount of damage perpetrated in the early days has been in part the fault of the Corporations in taking too much upon themselves. We do not believe that these arguments are valid. On the contrary, we feel that the Corporations have been considerate in their public relations and that their promotion of voluntary organizations has helped to create a good spirit among the tenants. It is very likely that the first wave of damage would have been greater and more prolonged if less encouragement had been given to voluntary work.

REFERENCES

[1]*Lord Hervey's Memoirs*, **ii**, p. 134.

[2]HAMMOND, J. L. & BARBARA (1930), *The Age of the Chartists*, p. 8, London: Longmans.

[3]PAPER BY J. O. MAY, *Trans. nat. Ass. Promotion Soc. Sc.*, **i**, 407.

[4]RUSSELL, J. B. (Memorial Volume) (1905): *Public Health Administration in Glasgow*, Glasgow: Maclehose.

[5]DE TOCQUEVILLE, ALEXIS (1945): *Democracy in America*, Vol. II, p. 133, New York: Knopf.

[6]MACKENZIE, NORMAN: *The New Towns*, Fabian Research Series No. 172.

[7]Ministry of Housing and Local Government (1956): *Moving from the Slums*, London: H.M.S.O.

[8]YOUNG, M. & WILLMOTT, P. (1957): *Family and Kinship in East London*, London: Routledge & Regan Paul.

Chapter 15

THE MEANING AND SCOPE
OF A PUBLIC HEALTH SERVICE

Many definitions and concepts of 'health' have been put forward, and it is customary, if not always wise, to begin a study of the subject with a series of definitions. In many cases it might be better to explore the confines of the subject first, and only then attempt to define the content and delimit the boundaries. In some instances what may be called a working definition is adopted. This is commonly a brief description, and is regarded as a useful guide to the reader. At any rate, the Constitution of the World Health Organization has set out on its remarkable career with a definition, or rather, a series of principles which are declared to be 'basic to the happiness, harmonious relations and security of all peoples'. The first clause runs as follows:

Health is a state of complete physical, mental and social well-being, and not merely the absence of disease or infirmity.

The remaining principles have a dynamic quality, stating the goals to be aimed at and the difficulties in the path to achievement. It is a fine statement, leading to the conclusion that the objective of the World Health Organization 'shall be the attainment by all peoples of the highest possible level of health'. This is a noble ideal, stated fully and expressed with force and sincerity. Yet the very heart of the definition leads one to question whether health is best described as a 'state'. One of the most vigorous definitions I have ever heard came from a remark made by a member of my staff who was responsible for student welfare. She said, 'What I mean by health is to get up every morning with eagerness to meet the challenge of the day's work.' There is something so mobile about this that one feels the contrasting listlessness of a state of complete physical, mental and social well-being.

Lord Radcliffe added to this comment in his fine book 'The Problem of Power', says:—

It is enervation of soul, an abdication of personal responsibility of judgment, that we have to fear. It does not come about because evil men set out to corrupt society: it comes about because the majority of members of society will always beg not to be required to keep themselves in training. And the whole pressure of the democratic State is in favour of giving them what they want. Modern life is lived as an essay in public relations. Facts themselves begin to matter less and less: all that matters is the way to put the thing. Persons themselves begin to matter less and less: all that matters is the kind of show they give. The spread of education has given most people the apparatus of criticism: what it has not always given them is the knowledge how to use their machine for an end that is not merely trivial or destructive. Yet criticism is essentially a method of appreciation. It has no necessary connection with the awful luxuries of contempt or condemnation. Uncontrolled by any positive wish to appreciate, criticism becomes nothing but the great escapist mechanism of modern culture. It is Mr. Everyman's excuse for not bothering.[1]

So it is with the practice of health. When the concept is static and materialistic, there is no sense of striving, no seeking to achieve a true balance between man and his environment—and this is what health means: 'to strive, to seek, to find, and not to yield.'?

Before the present century public health practice, even in the relatively advanced countries, had few functions; and most of them were concerned with preventing the spread of communicable diseases. In the earlier days, until the creation of a statutory service, this meant the attempt to block the passage of the great epidemics from a country of prevalence to the 'homeland', that is, the country which was feverishly seeking protection from invasion of pestilence. This sporadic activity in the presence of a grave menace of disaster is not preventive medicine but, as Winslow ingeniously put it, defensive medicine. It is a kind of fear reaction, and is generally too little and too late. 'When the plague was hot and furious, every man was holy and repentant; but with the slaking of the one came the forgetfulness of the other.'[2]

The next stages in health progress, in the older countries at least, were mainly associated with environmental sanitation. In most countries this had two aspects, the protection of the worker at his job by providing for reasonable working conditions and safety from obvious dangers, such as fire. This urgency arose on account of the sudden growth of the industrial system and the immediate hazards to workers who were at the mercy of uncontrolled industrial competition.

When we come to the present century we find that the emphasis on public health practice is steadily turning from environmental to personal and community care. An immense amount of functional activity has been added to the duties of the health officer, including such varied subjects as child care, the health of the ageing, and many other elements of public health which are predominantly social in character. In spite of the great enlargement of the field of his endeavour, we have to remind ourselves that one of the prime duties of the health officer is still unchanged in scope and responsibility. As the Romans said: *Caveant consules . . . ne quid respublica detrimenti caperet.* In spite of all the advances in scientific medicine, especially in the field of communicable diseases, the inescapable first duty of the health officer, wherever he be located, is to see that his community come to no harm. In view of this, he is not so much concerned with the niceties of diagnosis, especially if it is tied up with elaborate laboratory equipment, as with the simple duties of elementary protection. The sick man, perhaps a passenger on a ship from the Orient, may be suffering from a simple infection such as measles, to which he has in fact been exposed; but the function of the health officer is not to arrive at a final diagnosis after waiting patiently for the appropriate tests to be carried out and reported on Form 23/b. His duty is to take no avoidable risk, and his immediate answer in this case would be: 'Open a ward in the smallpox unit at once, and admit this patient for isolation, observation and treatment. In the meantime all contacts must be vaccinated, including nurses and staff members who can't show records of having been done within two years'.

This is rather a commonplace example, but the same principle applies to all matters concerning communicable disease and to other dangers liable to spread through the people: the escape of gas, the possibility of infected milk supply, the house that shows sudden cracks in the wall, or the dumping by accident of some noxious material on the public highway. The price of safety is vigilance—but by whom? It is no answer to say that certain measures of public safety are the function of certain technical experts. It is essential to know what experts are concerned. The answer to this problem has been stated with great ability and clarity by David Lilienthal:

'The unification of various technical skills', he says of TVA, 'was a central part of our task, as indeed it is a central problem in modern life. The skills are not self-co-ordinating . . . The breadth of TVA's undertaking itself made it imperative that we seek out the kind of experts who preferred to work as a part of a unified program. But even at best it is not easy for each specialist to appraise the relative importance of his own task as part of the whole picture, or its importance as compared with the tasks in some other technical branch. In fact, the desperate part of the problem, as many people have observed, is the realization of how rarely these different groups of specialists seem to care about anything beyond their own specialties.

This is not to say that specialists are narrow human beings. It is understandable that concentration and pre-occupation with a particular phase of a problem breeds impatience with anything not directly in the line of vision. The more conscientious and excited the specialist is about soil chemistry, metallurgy, fish and wild life, or statistical methods, the more likely he is to see all else as an adjunct.

It is an ironic fact that the very technical skills which are ostensibly employed to further the progress of men, by the intensity of their specialization, create disunity rather than order and imperil the whole success of their common objective. Resources cannot be developed in unity until each technologist has learned to subordinate his expertness to the common purpose, has come to see the region and its problems 'in its entirety'. . .

It was apparent to us, in the case I have described, that, at first look, at least one or more of the interests were in conflict. Differences of this kind could not be intelligently settled merely by compromise between the various technicians' views, a variation of the trader's 'splitting the difference'. But they had to be settled; a decision had to be made. Relative dollar cost was only one factor to be considered. The final question was always this: looking at the situation as a whole, and not merely at the professional or technical standards of any one or several of the specialized interests, what course of action would yield the best results *as judged by the common purpose*, the goal of the whole undertaking—the well-being of the people of the region? . . . The decisions made in many such reservoir cases are certainly not beyond question for their wisdom, but this at least is clear: they are products of a new kind of thinking. The problem was studied as a single problem.

With time, the barbed-wire fences began to come down within the TVA, the fences between the fields of special knowledge put up to keep one specialist out of the other fellow's domain and keep him in his own, barriers so characteristic of present-day science, of education, of engineering, even of theology. The TVA experts, themselves convinced of the value of combining their special judgments into a unified conclusion, soon developed workable methods of teamwork. It began to be taken more and more for granted (although 'backsliding' was, of course, not unknown) that expertness is not an end in itself, and that each skill is only one part of the unity of knowledge necessary to do the job of developing and conserving resources.

The common moral purpose of benefit to the people, by dint of observation and participation, came to be as real to the experts as some highly technical procedure had always been. They welcomed the chance to broaden their view of their own special fields and to relate them to other areas of knowledge.[3]

It is no answer to say that a particular risk lies outside the scope of the health officer. All matters that affect, or may affect, the health of the people, either within the area or without, are in his province. All public departments, no matter what their primary relation is, are within the scope of the health department so long as a risk to health is involved. The digging of a tunnel for the provision of a subway or a water supply*; a theatre or a public hall not sufficiently provided with a means of escape in the event of fire, or contributing to the danger of panic in the event of overcrowding—all these are *public health* risks, however much they have been safeguarded by law and regulation. The health officer cannot take cover under the reputed functions of another department in the case of disaster.

There are other aspects of this principle, the most important being that the health officer should be given time and opportunity to learn what is happening in his area, and have a real chance of personal inspection. He will know little about reality if he is perpetually confined to his office desk. A similar principle applies to the family doctor: if he does not know what the family and home background and the working conditions of his patients are, he is not a good family doctor.

* Cf. Croydon epidemic of typhoid.

As early as 1824 Gordon Smith gave an admirable definition of public health practice as 'the application of medical knowledge to the benefit of man in his social state'.[4] In 1883 the same term was defined by an expert as 'that branch of sanitary science which concerns the physical conditions of communities. It embraces a consideration of the various influences operating upon society, whether for its material good or its actual deterioration, with the view of extending the former and preventing or ameliorating, as far as possible, the latter'.[5] It will be observed that here the emphasis has been placed on environment.

One of the most informative descriptions of the functions of public health practice is to be found in a Minute of the English Board of Health, published in 1855 under the Public Health Act of 1848. It is of particular interest as being the first official statement related to the first Act of Parliament on this subject.

> 1. *The officer of health* is appointed—first, in order that through him the local sanitary authority may be duly informed of such influences as are acting against the healthiness of the population of his district, and of such steps as medical science can advise for their removal: secondly, to execute such special functions as may devolve upon him by the statute under which he is appointed; and thirdly, to contribute to the general stock of knowledge with regard to the sanitary condition of the people and to the preventable causes of sickness and mortality which, when collected, methodised, and reported to Parliament by the General Board of Health, may guide the Legislature in the extension and amendment of sanitary law.

The Minute then goes on to discuss in detail the day-to-day duties of the health officer, noting in particular that 'he will make himself familiar with the natural and acquired features of the place, with the social and previous sanitary state of the people, and with all its existing provisions for health.'

When we come to the application of these excellent suggestions, the real position was all too frequently as described in Smith's Manual of 1873: 'The Legislature has made abundant provision . . . but has *not* made it compulsory on the local authority.'[6] Indeed, the tragedy of the nineteenth century health service in England—which has been widely copied by the developing countries in the twentieth century—is that it was unable to act effectively. The central authority had powers which at first it had not educated the local authorities in using, and later it lost interest in even trying to use them. Even in the present age, in most of the industrialized countries, the central authority has been slow to wrath and abundant in mercy in its dealings with proprietary interests. Indeed, much of the urge to progress in health and housing came from the larger local authorities and battered against a reluctant central body. Happily, in recent years there have been increasing signs of co-operation between central and local authorities in the interests of the public health.

In discussing the expressions commonly used in relation to the health of the people, we have to refer to the meaning of the term 'principles'. A detailed consideration of preventive medicine and hygiene would occupy many volumes, because the application of these principles is concerned with the whole way of life. So the term, as used here, must refer to fundamental motives for action, and to the ideas which guide people consciously to a particular course of action. One of the essential principles of hygiene is to provide all the conveniences for healthy living. The environment is the framework which supports the life of the community, just as the house is the physical setting for the home. It is, of course, possible to discover healthy living without conveniences, and a clean bright home in the midst of a slum—but it does not follow that a bad environment is a school for virtue, or that amenities undermine the efforts of committees and individuals towards a healthy way of life—in spite of all that is said about 'the affluent society'. This has been shown again and again in public health practice: those who have experience of infant health centres know that they strengthen the self-reliance of the mothers who attend them. A more recent illustration of the same principle is manifest in the provision of family allowances, translating into practice a proposal made by William Pitt a hundred and sixty years ago:

> Let us make relief in cases where there are a number of children a matter of right and honour, instead of a ground for approbrium and contempt. This will make a large family a blessing, and not a curse; and this will draw a proper line of distinction between those who are able to provide for themselves by their labour, and those who, having enriched their country with a number of children, have a claim upon its assistance and support.[7]

It might be fair to say, then, that the first principle of health practice is the assurance of physical and economic opportunity for healthy living, without which the daily struggle of the great mass of men and women, especially in the less developed countries, is of no avail.

The second principle, which has been accepted in the advanced communities, is that, given this opportunity, the people are educated to *enjoy* healthy living, both as individuals and as members one of another. Much has been said and written during the past few years about education for health, but in many countries practical application still lags far behind knowledge.

The third principle depends upon a right conception of the meaning of health. Hitherto there has been much confusion of thought between the idea of health on the one hand and absence of disease on the other. Even yet we are not sure of our ground. In England the National Health Service Act of 1946 uses the expressions 'health service' and 'health centre' where the context evidently requires 'medical service' and 'medical care centre'. This is doubly unfortunate, because it bewilders the public mind about the true meaning of health, and it implies that 'medical care' is a less eligible term. In point of fact advances in medical care offer every reason at the present time for pride of achievement, and their positive contribution to health is of the utmost value. Further, the modern conception of the hospital as a centre for the restoration of health brings medical care into battle array by the side of the public health services, instead of apparent conflict.

This leads to the establishment of a fourth principle of health practice: that, in order to promote health, we must study with great care the causes of sickness. Until comparatively recently our statistical enquiries have been devoted largely to mortality and its causes, and valuable information has been gleaned from such figures. But today, both in industry and elsewhere, expert workers are concentrating their attention on the broader aspects of ill health, a great part of which is not represented in the records of death. The expression 'social medicine' indicates, not a new discovery in medical science, but a new attitude to sickness. It lays a just emphasis on the social factors involved in ill-health, and points clearly to the need for the study of man in his environment, that is, against the background of his family, his food, his house, and his work and play.

STANDARDS

There is a natural tendency to discuss health service in terms of an ideal to be aimed at. When we come down to the world as it is, it is only too clear that our standards represent what is feasible in a given country at a given time. Essentially this amounts to the study of background, and estimates of what is possible. Background factors, such as climate, social and economic security; environment such as water supply, temperature, and the nature of the ground for building and drainage; local building and other materials; personal factors relating to minimum standards including education, political situation, government, religion, custom and tradition. Such things as world minimum standards could be readily adopted in a large number of cases. The obvious examples are pharmaceutical products, nutrition, housing and town planning.

It is of course easy to talk about standards; but it is hard to secure their application under conditions so diverse as are found even in a single country. On the other hand, we have some knowledge of values, freedom from bias, and integrity, and at least the elements can be taught. To take a few simple illustrations, the nature of a building to be used as a home varies from one area to another, but there are certain basic features, from which a selection could be made anywhere. Many of these have been well brought forward in 'The basic principles of healthy housing', and in the many booklets of advice issued in England by the Ministry of Health. Some excellent accounts of the principles of housing in the tropics have also been published, notably by Fry. The real difficulty is not to establish standards but to see that they are obeyed. It is in this respect that the promotion of international standards is particularly effective.

The function of international organizations can be laid out in terms of definition and possible goals. For those which are based on national interests, the first step is to extend the relevant parts of national effort into the international sphere, at the same time strengthening the national counterpart. The earliest duty is to make sure of a proper interest and effort among the nations, and to avoid the risks due to the showering of favours in money and personnel on any special group. The temptation to do this is very great, for several reasons: firstly, because it is easy to assist those who are eager to be helped and ready to co-operate in every detail. Secondly, it is tempting to choose personnel from countries known to be advanced in teaching or research. And thirdly, the areas which already possess laboratories and equipment, organized services, good transport and similar amenities seem most likely to produce quick and satisfactory results.

For all types of international organization there exists the perpetual risk of becoming, as it were, supra-national, by taking on functions which national governments ought to carry out themselves. The temptation to supersede, rather than to assist, local and national effort, has nearly always a boomerang effect, and is invariably the wrong policy. The only right international policy is to help people to build up their own services and to rely on their own trained staff, always provided that the assistance given by the international organization is adequate for the purpose in hand. No one knows this better than the international agencies themselves, and they are often misunderstood in consequence by those who are in a hurry. Patience is one of the supreme virtues of international work.

Value and Urgency

When all that has been said above has been accepted, and the international agency is ready to give its help to a willing and eager recipient nation, there remain a number of 'obstinate questionings' of a deeper kind. For example, nothing can be more urgent than the mass eradication of a communicable disease from a people, or the cleansing of their streets, the creation of homes, and the planning of public health services. Yet there are other values to be weighed in the balance of national well-being. Simple examples are the preservation of natural beauty, the conservation of soil, the planning of towns worthy of a great community, the construction of noble buildings, and the promotion of learning. One of the highest functions of non-governmental organizations is to take these and other values into account, and to cherish them in a bleak world.

There appeared recently in one of our principal newspapers the following letter:

PAINTINGS OR PEOPLE?

Assessing values in the world today

" Sir,

In 1960, World Refugee Year, what painting is worth over £128,000? What are the true values of the world today?"

Another application of the principles of values can be illustrated in the planning of towns and cities, and their public buildings. In this function it is important that our assessment should not confuse civic value with civic urgency. Nothing can be more urgent than the health of the people, which involves the lives of men and women; or industrial and commercial prosperity, on which depend the livelihood of the citizens. Without these supports the city would founder, and all its other achievements would sink into the past. So it is easy to understand why many people seem to think that the only sound policy is to build, as they would put it, from the ground—by concentrating all their sympathy, effort, and expenditure on public health, elementary education, industrial organization, and the like, and 'by refusing to lift a finger to organize and equip higher education or to found museums and art galleries, or to rear stately public buildings and so forth, until every citizen is well-fed, well-housed, and decently clad.'[8] Now I quote the following as *the MacCunn Principle,* because it was expressed so clearly by my old friend, Professor John MacCunn, more than fifty years ago. And I believe it to hold its truth today, in *any* country, and especially those which are on the threshold of development. With regard to those who hold to the idea of serving physical necessities first he says: 'Nor is this an ideal of which anyone need be ashamed; for it is often motivated by a depth of sympathy with hardship and suffering which commands respect. But it is a mistaken ideal nonetheless. It views the growth of a city mechanically as if it were the building of a house, of which the foundations must be complete before any superstructure can be reared thereon. But the fact stands otherwise. A city is an organism. And this being so, its friends and administrators can no more afford to neglect the less urgent, but not less valuable, elements of civic life than the father of a family can postpone the education of his sons until their bodies have reached maturity. Even as, in the growing boy, the tiny shoots of intellectual promise must, on penalty of the impoverishment of a lifetime, be vigilantly fostered, so in the larger organism the less urgent, less immediately necessary ends and interests, which may by and by render it famous, must be recognized and encouraged long before the city has become great in industry and commerce. . . . The besetting danger lies in the opposite direction. It is so easy for the utilities which are obvious, tangible, necessary, urgent, to be pushed to the front, and for the spiritualities, *the goods of the soul*, as the Greeks called them, to be ignored or thrust into the background.'

There are examples of magnificent temples and monuments, theatres, libraries, and great public buildings all over the world. One does not only have to seek in Greece and Rome, Egypt or India, to see the finest works of man. The first point is whether they represent real civic values today; and the second matter is whether they genuinely stand for a sense of common enjoyment, or is it in danger of being lost? In their fine book, 'The Age of the Chartists', the Hammonds suggested that, even among the slaveries and cruelties of the ancient world, these graces of ownership by the people went far to mitigate the harshness of the world of men. Even in our own time there are great examples of civic values.

The dilemma of civic need and civic value is serious, and it cannot be stabilized in a balance by any simple rule. An interesting and remarkable example of this dilemma arose in the English City of Coventry, which had been desperately damaged by enemy attack. One of the outstanding misfortunes was the destruction of its great Citizen's Cathedral. Some years after the war the question of rebuilding the cathedral came into prominence, and a licence to carry out the work was requested from the government. A deputation from the City Council then approached the Minister (Sir David Eccles), objecting to the proposal on the ground that other and more important social buildings were needed. The Minister, in his reply, observed that his duty was to enquire whether the Cathedral could be rebuilt without undue interference with other work in progress or ready to start. He was satisfied that many beautiful materials would in fact be made by fine craftsmen who had suffered greatly since the war, and that the building ought to go on. And he added:

'I hope that my decision will be accepted on wider grounds.

The Cathedral is not a building which concerns Coventry and Coventry alone. The echo of bombs which destroyed your city was heard round the world. We cannot tell how many people are waiting in this country and abroad for this church to rise and prove that English traditions live again after the blitz. The threat of far worse destruction is with us today, demoralizing and corrupting our thoughts. We have never had a greater need for acts of faith.'

REFERENCES

[1] RADCLIFFE, LORD (1952): *The Problem of Power,* Glasgow: Collins.

[2] HOLINSHED, 1580. *Chronicles.*

[3] LILIENTHAL, David E. (Chairman, Tennessee Valley Authority) (1944): *TVA Democracy on the March,* p. 66, New York and London: Harper Brothers.

[4] SMITH, JOHN GORDON (1824), *The Principles of Forensic Medicine.*

[5] and [6] SMITH's *Manual of Hygiene,* 1873.

[7] WILLIAM PITT, *Speech in House of Commons.*

[8] MACCUNN, JOHN (1911): *Ethics of Social Work,* Liverpool University Press.

Chapter 16

MEDICAL CARE TOMORROW

The pattern of medical care tomorrow will be woven out of these strands of today:

1. Advances in the treatment of manifest disease.
2. Discovery arising from research and good luck.
3. The study of the epidemiology of health and sickness.
4. Efficient organisation for the prevention and care of sickness, in the individual and in the community.
5. Education in medical, nursing and allied disciplines.

All statements of this kind involve selection, and it might be a useful exercise to calculate how many strands have been omitted. In getting a right perspective it does us no harm to look back over half a century or so, and to find a measure to stretch into the future.

I wish I could take you back to the wards of a great teaching hospital as I first saw it 50 years ago. Let us do a quick bed round, first in the female ward.

Here is a young woman who is a clerk in a store. What you notice at a glance is the curious pallor of her skin and shadowed eyes, although her cheeks are well rounded. She will tell you that she gets breathless easily, and that her feet swell in the evening. There is no doubt about the diagnosis, and the girl is being vigorously treated with iron, which blackens her teeth and makes her even more constipated. In the course of a few weeks her haemoglobin rises to a reasonable level, and she goes back to work, drinks more tea, eats more white bread and jam, and sweet cakes and soon returns to her former state of chlorosis.

What was wrong with us? Well, we allowed her to get the disorder, largely from lack of education in healthful living. Of course, there were many contributing causes, such as bad housing, tight corsets, long hours of standing, lack of exercise and, above all, poor feeding. But that's not all: we sent her back to the same conditions that produced her disease, without any attempt to follow up; we did not offer her the help she so desperately needed, or check her progress from week to week. And worse still, the fact that there were masses of girls suffering from the same condition did not automatically operate the wheels of research.

In the next bed is a young girl of 16. As we approach there is a look of apprehensive terror on her face, and yet she makes no movement. Her wrists are bandaged and there is a sickly smell around the bed—of oil of wintergreen. She has acute rheumatic fever, and a touch from a careless hand is agony to her. Under care she will soon be free from pain, but in the meantime she is busy manufacturing the disease that we see in the next bed in its full development.

Here is a young married woman who had her first baby a few months ago. She sits up in bed leaning on stacked pillows. At rest she seems fairly comfortable but looks old and tired for her years, and slight exertion makes her struggle for breath. The physician tells his students to listen for the rough murmur just before each heartbeat. She is not going to have any more babies.

Who is to watch and help this young woman during the long losing battle after she is discharged? And who is studying the origins of this disease in the community and the means of prevention? Who has the responsibility for collecting the records from hundreds of hospitals and so studying the epidemiology of the disease? Who is on guard against its reappearance, armed with full information?

In the three neighbouring beds, we find rather older women, all suffering from the same disease but in different phases. The first has a difficult, short cough that catches her painfully in the side. Her temperature rose to 104° F. last night. The second woman has been struggling for five days against increasing breathlessness, and by now her colour is dusky and she no longer cares what happens. Occasionally they give her a whiff of oxygen from a clumsy mask. The third woman lies low in a state of mumbling exhaustion. Late last night it did not seem possible that she could survive, and then the miracle happened —the crisis. Appetite and strength will soon return, and everyone takes heart again.

These three women were suffering from a disease that has now lost its terrors. All the same, the pneumococcus has friends and relatives among the organisms. In many ways he has been a good friend himself to the aged and has smoothed many a passage to death. Is it right that modern medicine should cancel his more kindly services and replace them with suffering that has no purpose but to prolong suffering? Might we not say with the poet:

> Vex not his ghost: O, let him pass! He hates him
> That would upon the rack of this tough world
> Stretch him out longer.

And so I could go on, past that deep-eyed girl dying of miliary tuberculosis and the old woman with a persistent ulcer on her foot and a load of sugar in her urine.

Now let us turn to the male ward, for time is short, and the Art is long. Here the picture is altered to some extent by the presence of a selection of arterial disorders, including various stages of aneurysm and some of the now obsolete forms of late syphilis. Duodenal ulcer is represented, but not more frequently than pernicious anemia or carcinoma of the head of the pancreas. No one hears of carcinoma of the respiratory tract.

What has happened during the 50 years? We are familiar with the great changes resulting from the use of the antibiotics and with the striking advances in protection by inoculation. The use of vitamins and mineral salts has been immensely extended, and sometimes their abuse. Surgery has won its triumphs also, and innumerable techniques have been improved or introduced for the first time. All these, and I have quoted only a few, are on the credit side of the balance.

There are other features, more subtle and less prominent in the public mind. The first that strikes me is the enormous improvement in hospital administration. Half a century ago the hospital was more or less heavily tainted with the stigma of poverty, and at its best, the services it rendered were acts of charity rather than applications of science and skill. One of the principal difficulties was the inaccessibility of the great specialised hospitals to many of those who were in need of the highest skills. Another was the all but total lack of co-operation between one unit and another, and therefore the unnecessary duplication of expensive equipment, with equally noteworthy gaps in the supplies for everyday care.

Today it is realised that the hospital administrator is a trained officer who has knowledge of policy, construction and services, and who can see them whole. It is obvious that the advance and unavoidable narrowing of medical specialism must lead to a corresponding limitation of his vision of the hospital as a whole. This is not a matter for complaint but for understanding. The very skill that has created the specialty must limit the range because the higher focal power is accompanied by a narrower field of vision.

Now, this growth in administrative skill and experience ought not to be linked with a narrow field of operation. When physicians become more specialised, they must necessarily enter into more consultation with their colleagues in neighbouring disciplines. In the same way, hospital administration must develop the qualities of the team, both in relation to the single unit and to co-operation over a region. In other words, in any hospital region there should be an administrative faculty that will be able to deal with all types of medical care, not in one unit alone, but in the area as a whole.

Just as we know that A.B. deals with orthopaedics and C.D. with medical rehabilitation, so we must be sure that one administrator is primarily responsible for certain services for the benefit of the sick. This grouping does not detract from the responsibility of each administrator in a hospital, but it does impose on him some special obligations in which he is expected to exercise special skill. How is this to be accomplished in practice? It can be done only in one way—by voluntary agreement. And there must be frequent staff meetings for consultation.

On the stricter side of medical care, we should really be concerned about: (1) the conditions that cut off life in its prime; (2) the disasters that curtail life in the richness of its experience; (3) the conditions and disabilities that limit the fullness of life and health through mental or physical disability, and (4) the strategy of prevention.

Under conditions that cut off life in its prime, we have still to include tuberculosis and the acute communicable diseases, many of which are not yet conquered, or are at least smouldering. The overwhelming majority of them, including tuberculosis, should be 'in the bag' in the course of the next half century. It is in this group that the greatest advances have already been made, and they hold the highest promise, the major tropical disease, such as malaria and yaws, not being forgotten.

R

In the second group—disasters that curtail life in the richness of its experience—we have the dark shadows of cancer and the cardio-vascular diseases. For one reason or another, the problem of unfair wear and tear has come increasingly before the technically advanced peoples, and, perhaps in similar categories, the mental disorders and the psychoneuroses. We are making some progress in this field, but not enough.

Perhaps the whole question of this second group will have to be re-examined and dealt with by a completely fresh approach through the social sciences and by a reappraisal of the physical effects of undue strain in the ways of living. Our present snatches at the disorders of the circulation and at the more obscure associations of mental ill health simply will not do; we shall have to broaden the whole issue of research to comprise the social sciences, and particularly social psychology and anthropology.

The third group—conditions and disabilities that limit the fullness of life and health through mental or physical disability—is less well defined, but it includes the handicapped, whether the disability arises from genetic causes, disease, or accident. Unhappily, an increasing number of physical disabilities are due to avoidable accidents at home or on the road, and our methods of prevention are often feeble and sluggish.

One of the first duties of medical care is a realistic attack on the avoidable disabilities. The next duty is to man and to hold the lines against the diseases of childhood, and especially to be on the watch against new encroachments. In dealing with communicable disease, the price of safety is eternal vigilance. In this respect one should notice that the criteria adopted by the health officer are different from those of the clinician and the bacteriologist.

In other words, the first duty of the health officer is to protect the public safety. He is not primarily concerned with the niceties of diagnosis.

In this sphere, however, there are two schools of thought, and their action will be of great moment during the coming half century. The first group says: 'We must keep up our pressure all along the line'; the other group, 'No, we ought to have a well-thought-out strategy, and we ought to attack, using all our resources, at the point where we are likely to secure the maximum results.'

The adherents of the second group, for example, would concentrate on world tuberculosis, in the hope of delivering a
knockout blow. Some of the pitched battles against malaria are
a fair illustration of this method, and both campaigns would
have to be on a vast scale and would involve serious sacrifices in
other branches of medical care. You cannot launch an all-out
offensive against a number of targets at the same time, and you
will be lucky, if you succeed in 'holding' actions elsewhere, when
you are dealing with tuberculosis. On the other hand, the effect
of a single blow might be so devastating that the sacrifice would
be worthwhile, and in the long run an international triumph.

There is another answer, of course: if we devoted a relatively
small part of the money spent on war and preparation for war,
the mighty campaign against disease would be a human
triumph, and the cause of peace and international co-operation
could be won on a single issue.

For the third category—the curtailment of useful life in its
fullness—no such all-out campaign is needed. The problem of
the next half century is essentially one of scientific research. We
must tackle, for example, with all the weapons at our disposal,
the immense problem of cancer—genetic, organismal, or a
response to prolonged irritation—or a combination of these.
We must study the vegetative reprisals against the long domi-
nation of sex: the more primitive urge for mere tissue survival
when the sexual function has failed, through age or disorder, to
supply the necessary controls. Cancer is like a civilised country
in which the failure of government control has led inexorably to
anarchy, and the main characteristic of the anarchy is the
pathetic attempt to achieve mere group survival at the expense
of the body politic.

It is true that neither tyranny nor cancer arises in sound
constitutions; there must be an outward irritant such as political injustice, poverty, and the like, in the one case, and certain
external irritants in the other—and for these tobacco, certain
oils and smog have been blamed. But once the process gets into
motion, the irritated part will destroy the individual. It is at
any rate noteworthy that most cancers show themselves at a
time when the sexual function is weakening; it is also at a time
when irritants have had an opportunity of becoming well
established and are able to show their characteristic reactions.

This is, of course, a fanciful analogy; but in our circumstances we should not fail to pursue shadows. We may find unexpected substance lying around. And after all, man is the shadow of a dream.

In the cardiovascular diseases, we must guard against excessive wear and tear. Ordinary wear may be regarded as natural, like death, but it is a warning sign against overactivity. If we accept the compliment that coronary thrombosis is mainly a disorder of the intelligent hard worker, this does not preclude us from a careful scientific investigation of its exciting causes. The intelligent perhaps drink more coffee than the dull, but certainly they take less exercise. There are many possibilities to be studied, with human controls.

There is not a great deal to be said about the disability group; in some ways they are the most disappointing of all, because one part is associated with genetic causes, which we are doing our best to multiply; and the other is chiefly due to accident, hustle and bustle, which we increase day after day. We can at least give time and thought to such conditions as cerebral palsy or the aftereffects of poliomyelitis, and we can constantly improve the salvage work of surgery.

Our fourth subject is concerned with the strategy of prevention. What are to be the functions of the hospital of the future? In this connection, we must remember that the cost of medical care is going to rise with the increasing complexity of treatment. This is both right and inevitable, but it means that we shall have to conserve our slender resources for those who stand in greatest need of these expensive services.

We can no longer afford to maintain in a hospital bed a patient who does not require, and continue to require, highly specialised or urgent treatment. Waiting, care and maintenance, or convalescence in an acute general hospital is a costly anachronism. And this applies equally to mental hospitals. The turnover of patients in the great hospitals has increased, but we are still hardly touching the fringe of the problem, partly because we have so far failed to design, still less to provide, satisfactory alternative accommodation and staffing for those who are not in immediate need of specialised treatment, or for patients who for the time being require only diagnostic facilities.

The simple truth is this: our acute hospitals must have a swift and effective exchange system through which patients can be transferred in the twinkling of an eye from more costly to less costly accommodation, without any loss of care. The less expensive type will have to be on the spot, and not in some remote seaside lodging. We do not keep patients in operating rooms longer than is absolutely necessary, but we shall have to learn that every bed in an acute general hospital is an operating room. To put the matter in another way, the concept of a well directed and comfortable hostel for those who are not, in a medical sense, undergoing operations is urgent.

The Mayo Clinic in Rochester, Minn., has already gone far in this direction, and a number of other hospitals have made progress along similar lines. In many countries, however, there has been no attempt to follow the lead. The cost of construction and the total operating cost should be less than half that of an acute hospital, and the apparatus for diagnosis is quite different. The hostel will also have to provide temporary residence for visitors and waiting relatives as well as for patients, with simple hotel charges to cover food and lodging.

Changes of this kind can be effective only if we are prepared to revolutionise our ideas for the design of general, special and mental hospitals. Most sick people are much more mobile than we used to believe, and we know that movement has some real advantages. I have to add sadly that some of our legal colleagues need education in this respect, as they seem to regard all movement with suspicion.

In this connection one of the most important collaborators of the hospital director is the engineer. Many of the essential problems of handling the sick are associated with lifting and moving, and there is no doubt that, under guidance, the engineer could give us a vast amount of assistance. In fact, he could be the master magician of movement in the hospital and its younger brother, the hostel.

Movement means bringing the patient to the dressing room, the eating room, and the toilet, as well as to the x-ray and other specialised departments. All beds must move, and the problem resolves itself into engineering methods for making movement pleasant and easy. When the atrocious bedpan has been properly consigned to oblivion, except for the quite exceptional case, then we shall have eased the work of the skilled staff beyond measure, and the hospital life of the sick will have become much more bearable. We have now opened the doors of many of the mental hospitals. The time has come to open the doors of the general hospitals.

So, too, the engineer will help us materially in the reduction of noise and glare, two of the greatest bugbears of the sick. He will redesign lavatory accommodations to meet the real needs of the sick, in place of the present feeble imitation of the household system. The design of hospital toilets and lavatories has not been seriously thought about for a hundred years.

Hostels ought to be redesigned from the ground, and someone should offer a good prize for an imaginative plan. It should have the qualities of a good, but not extravagant, hotel, with wide doors for the movement of beds and, of course, bedside elevators, and appropriate moving stairways. These hostels are intended for sick people, and are not to be regarded as purely convalescent homes. They are, in fact, annexes of hospitals and are under their government, and of course the patients are wholly under their care. They are not to be confused with what have been known as 'home hospitals' under the care of general physicians, although they may well replace them, and become the meeting ground for the specialist, the general physician and the nurse.

I am not going to say much about hospital care as such. Until the concept of the hostel is fully established for both mental and physical patients, we are beating the air in vain. In the hospital of tomorrow, every bed will be specialised, and medical care will be an operation just as much as is surgical treatment. In a considerable number of cases, of course, the essential operative procedure will be skilled nursing, and in the hospital of tomorrow the registered nurse will have to devote all her time to her highly specialised work, free from the unwelcome interference of administrative or domestic duties.

Recent studies of nursing services have convinced me that it is a specialised profession and that the nurse can—and should—take the place of the doctor in many medical functions both in the home and in the hospital, and especially in the hostel.

The category of ward assistants, with a more practical training, should be introduced without delay, and a scheme of this kind would have a wide application throughout the world. The chief difficulties seem to be a fear of 'dilution' in the nursing profession on the one hand, and a want of clear thinking about the assistant's duties on the other. The training of the nurse would then be a full university course. The transition from assistant to nurse should be of the same order as transition from laboratory technician to scientist, through the acquisition of a qualification of university standard. On the other hand, I should regard the assistant in a hospital as a technician who requires a standard training of not less than two years, and sound practical experience in addition.

I must touch briefly on a further aspect of the strategy of prevention—the need for change in the structure of medical administration in this country. Most authorities agree that the basic requirement of a sound health service, in the broadest sense, is the closest possible link between home care, hospital care and the public health service. What can we devise tomorrow to replace our temporary structures by permanent building?

I personally hold the view that, in all forms of government administration, both central and local, the final responsibility should lie with the elected representatives of the people, and that the people should have a full opportunity, at intervals of not less than five years, of freely electing their chosen representatives.

Secondly, a changing social structure and, especially, the great increase of transportation facilities have rendered necessary a widening of the area of local government. This can now be done effectively without individual and communal responsibility being reduced. This change is necessary, but it should not be made because the wider area is an end in itself, or because it would disregard sentimental attachment to the conduct of affairs within the narrowest possible local limits.

Nearly a century and a half ago, Alexis de Tocqueville,[1] writing of the United States, said:

'However enlightened and however skilful a central power may be, it cannot of itself embrace all details of the existence of a great nation. . . . And, when it attempts to create and set in motion so many complicated springs, it must submit to a very imperfect result, or consume itself in bootless efforts. Centralisations succeeds more easily, indeed, in subjecting the external actions of men to a certain uniformity . . . and perpetuates a drowsy precision in the conduct of affairs which is hailed by the heads of the administration as a sign of perfect order . . . in short, it excels more in prevention than in action. Its force deserts it when society is to be disturbed or accelerated in its course; and if once the co-operation of private citizens is necessary to the furtherance of its measures, the secret of its importance is disclosed. Even while it evokes their assistance, it is on the condition that they shall act exactly as much as the government chooses, and exactly in the manner it appoints. . . . These, however, are not the conditions on which the alliance of the human will is obtained; its carriage must be free, and its actions responsible, or such is the constitution of man, the citizen had rather remain a passive spectator than an actor who can be relied upon, in schemes with which he is unacquainted.'

There is the case for local control in administration. Its effectiveness can be determined by two tests: (1) Do the men in the field have the power of decision? (2) Are the people and their local institutions actively participating in the enterprise?

To sum up: In medical care tomorrow the outstanding need is for unity of administration on the understanding that we can no longer go back to the small areas of local government that were sufficient for the simpler needs of the nineteenth and early twentieth centuries. It is widely admitted that larger governmental units are indispensable, and there is a good deal of agreement that an appropriate population for urban areas would be in the region of half a million. This would of course have to be modified for scattered rural communities, for transportation rather than population is the real test.

With a local governmental unit of about this size it should be possible to organise an effective service of medical care combined with public health, and so to create a national health service. Under such a scheme there would be a true public health service with a great deal of local autonomy and an opportunity for local initiative. Certain highly specialised services would be reserved to larger areas, as, for example, where university supervision was necessary. These services, however, although of great importance and often highly complicated and costly, offer no serious administrative obstacle.

I believe that the special value of medical care is to get as near the people as possible; to make the people feel that they are partners in the enterprise, and to build up a strong and efficient local administration. One of the planners of a great scheme of regional administration, the Tennessee Valley Authority, said: [2]

'There are of course many instances where the facts appear to support the claim that good administration of national concerns cannot be obtained through the co-operation of local agencies. Local politics, ineptitude, lack of interest and experience in public matters and in administration, brazen partisanship, even corruption—all these stand in the way. I am sure these hazards exist. But what are the alternatives?

'Fewer citizens participating in governmental administration. Less and less local community responsibility. More federal employees in the field armed with papers to be filled out and sent to Washington for processing, because only there is good administration possible. The progressive atrophy of citizen interest. An ever wider gulf between local communities and national government, between citizens and their vital public concerns.'

REFERENCES

[1] DE TOCQUEVILLE, A. (1945): *Democracy in America* (original edition, 1835), New York, Knopf.

[2] LILIENTHAL, D. E. (1944): *TVA Democracy on the March,* New York, Harper Brothers.

Chapter 17

OUT OF THE SHADOWS

It is difficult to be sure when the shadows began to fall, but the first intimation was during a journey by air. It was bright in the sunshine at 20,000 feet, but when I looked down on the fleecy clouds out of the corner of one eye, I was surprised to find them grey. The other eye was brought into use to confirm, and the brilliant white at once returned. A few trials showed that there was a marked difference between the two eyes— and so the long pilgrimage into the shadows began.

A few days later the ophthalmologist incriminated both lenses, but the one was in a very early stage, without real loss of sight for reading. 'I'll do the first eye any time,' said he, but I waited. It does not make sense to become incapacitated, when one eye is almost perfect. In this way the months passed, and the twilight fell so insidiously. A moment came when a reading glass had to be introduced to deal with newspaper type, and before long this awkward aid had to be extended to ordinary typescript, just nine months after the first recognition of cataract.

A few weeks later the stage of embarrassment was upon me: friends passing in the office corridors were not recognised. 'Have you noticed that M. is much less friendly than he used to be? Why, only yesterday he went past me in the corridor without so much as a nod, let alone a smile . . . seems to think a lot of himself these days.'

Between nine months and twelve the embarrassment grew apace, and the condition could no longer be concealed, because reading had become too difficult and even traffic on the crowded roads too dangerous. 'But why,' said Jane, 'Why should you want to conceal and enter into pretences, in an obviously disabling condition like cataract?' The answer is not so simple as it looks. The real trouble is that the condition is not obvious, as often as not, it has to be explained. And the mere explanation sounds as if it were designed to excite sympathy. 'So sorry not to recognise you, but you see, my eyes are rather feeble because of cataract.' This is not in fact convincing; it gives the other person an uncomfortable sense of having failed in the little courtesies of life: 'Oh, I'm sorry; of course I should have known.' Or again: 'Did you read that paper I sent along to you last week?' 'No, I couldn't manage it; you see, I have a catar-act.' 'Oh, I beg your pardon. Of course, I ought not to have sent it.' And so the slow estrangement grows between the victim and his surrounding world. He peers through the shadows and his isolation deepens the twilight. 'Lonely fellow, that M. Not up to his job, I think. Said to have some eye trouble, but if you ask me, I should say that he's just going slow.' Of course people don't really talk like that, or very few of them; but the suspicion grows in the darkening mind rather than in the outer world.

They why not go and have the thing out at once, and not wait for the other eye nor for the traditional ripening of the earlier cataract? In my case the superficial answer was easy. I was in a foreign land, and would be surrounded, in the dark day following operation, by kind attendants who could not easily interpret my needs. Nursing customs would be different from home, and perhaps even the surgical procedures unfami-liar. Would it be better to wait for the return home or to have the two eyes done at the same time? Were these the real reasons, or did something lie deeper, such as the fear of mutilation, or another primitive and irrational doubt. Or perhaps 'better to bear those ills we have than fly to others that we know not of . . .'

Then came the gracious and joyous invitation, and there was no longer any doubt. In a few weeks I had crossed the Atlantic and was waiting, with a great sense of calm, to see the surgeon. 'Well now,' said the assistant, after a thorough examination, 'Dr. X does not like to examine his patients until he has had plenty of time to study all the documents. Come back in about two hours' time.'

When I came back, I was thoroughly examined by one who obviously knew the whole story and that alone gave me further confidence. There was an air of quiet as he turned to me and folded his hands. 'Your cataracts are not far advanced,' he said, 'and in ordinary circumstances you might get along pretty well for months, perhaps as much as a year, without having anything done. But your reading is relatively poor, and I

imagine you depend on that for your day's work. (Pause) I
could of course do one eye, and you might enjoy a long period of
reasonable sight for reading. (Pause) Or I could deal with both
eyes, although one of them is at an early stage. An interval of
about two weeks would enable you to go around all the time
without having to depend on others to any extent, and of course
the balance of vision for reading. . . . But it is a long time since
you graduated in medicine, so we might have a look at this
model together.' And thereupon he produced a large-scale
model and showed simply and clearly, what it all meant. There
was no doubt in my mind, but we waited once more for a few
moments. 'I should like you to do both eyes,' I said. 'Very well,'
he replied, 'I'll do the right one at eleven o'clock tomorrow, and
the left a fortnight later.' And so it was, with unhurrying speed.

It is impossible to avoid a certain amount of nervous tension
in association with an eye operation, but when the hospital has
the right spirit, there is a sense of sharing with others which
takes away the sharpness of anxiety; and so it was here. We
were all in the fun, staff and patients alike, and isolation disappeared by magic. I suppose I ought to be more critical, especially in view of the large number of hospitals I have visited in my
time, but it was a very happy occasion, to be remembered
always. The spirit belongs to the hospital and not to any one
section or department, and it defies analysis. Ask a taxi driver
or a member of the police force about the hospital, and he
glows with pride. That is a good test. And what does it matter
in the long run, if the air-conditioner roars like a tempest or the
lavatory basin has a faucet that hits you between the eyes when
you try to have a wash? Now that I come to think of it, the coat
hangers were the real menace; they had a habit of digging
themselves into your eye at the critical moment when you were
reaching for that shirt. I suppose they would be kinder if they
were installed with their flat sides toward impatient patients.
But these are trivialities.

My wife Marjorie wrote to me quite often, and she has a
genius (denied to me) for making commonplace events sound
interesting. These letters were read to me day by day by a
sympathetic student nurse. When the time came for me to leave,
I thanked this nurse—very sincerely—for her help in reading
the letters and laboriously writing my replies. I ended by

saying 'And I shall miss you very much.' With a flash of Irish intuition she answered 'And I shall miss Marjorie something terrible.'

Well, the time came for discharge, and I went out into the hot, humid world with reluctance, although I was armed and well prepared. My glasses were of course of the blunderbuss type, and some six weeks had to go by before the definite fitting. These were adventurous days of trial and error, drenching sun and the patient search for shadow. I had not realised, in spite of telling, what an implacable enemy pursued me in the form of Glare, and no form of shade that I could find offered sufficient protection. Before long I made the fascinating discovery that, while the blind are (very properly) cared for by all who recognise their badge of a white stick, those that walk in the shadows have no such protection. This limitation applies especially to those who have no public functions to perform. They say to themselves half-consciously, when you ask them to guide you across the road or to the nearest taxi stand or bus top: 'Confound his cheek, how shall I get rid of this hanger-on?' As often as not they give a sort of grudging help—and then make themselves scarce as quickly as possible, to avoid further imposition. This is understandable enough, for the half-blind have no badge of claim, and no obvious need like a physically handicapped person.

There is a further point: that the weak-sighted want to do as much as they can for themselves and do not seem to need protection as a rule. And yet, shall I ever forget the experience of coming out of a store into the blazing sun and a temperature of 101°. Back I went into the store and asked a couple of customers to help me to get a taxi. 'Oh' said they, 'you just stand there on the sidewalk till a cab comes up.' So I went out again, and in a moment or two there was a movement by my side. It was the policeman on busy traffic duty at the crossroad. 'I see you're in trouble,' he said. 'Just take my arm and we'll go across into the shade. Where do you want to go?' And in three minutes a shrill whistle brought a cab to a standstill in front of me. A wave of the hand and he was back to his traffic problems, having first solved mine.

I had similar experiences with many of those who had some public duty to perform—railroad officials and waiters, hotel staff, and customs officer. 'Take a seat,' said one of them when I arrived exhausted at an airport of entry. 'Let me see your checks.' I gave him all the tickets I had, and he looked through them. 'I see your plane is due to leave for New York in half-an-hour. You haven't much time to get across.' Then he disappeared mysteriously, to return in a few minutes. 'It's all right,' he said, a little diffidently, 'I called the American Airline, and their plane is late, too. So you have an hour to spare. Don't hurry. Oh, by the way,' he continued almost at once, 'I had your baggage checked through while I was at it . . . no trouble at all. Good journey.'

At last the great awakening came. I had waited for a week after the final prescription had been made out, and now the time came to receive the glasses. Cautiously I put them on and turned from the optician's counter to the street. The sun was too strong for the sudden change, and, as in the Gospel story, I only saw 'men as trees walking.' The real miracle did not appear until the following morning, when I turned in the half-light and gazed at the dim, distorted room of the hotel. With anxious care I reached for the new glasses and put them on. Instantly every detail was clear, and I emerged from the shadows. . . . Eagerly I moved across the room to pick up the paper. It was true; the smallest print was clear as day.

Four months have gone by. What is the assessment? First, there is the physical condition of the eyes themselves, which have shown a steady improvement in balance and have more than fulfilled their promise of good vision, both near and far. My reading capacity is called 'agate' in England, and, I believe, 'point 5' in the United States. The main interest now rests on acquiring skill in overcoming the inevitable restriction of visual fields. Stiff-necked people had better avoid cataract, because width of vision no longer depends upon the sidelong glance, but on the speed and precision of head movements, both vertically and horizontally. One could make a pretty series of 'Rules for Aphakics' (what a horrible word!).* Shall we call them 'Aphakians?'

1. Leave your glasses where you can find them easily. This applies especially to the bedside at night. There are few things

* Aphakia is a condition in which the lens is absent from the dioptic system—Blakiston's New Gould Medical Dictionary.

more ridiculous than a sprawling aphakian searching for his 'windows to the world.'

2. Keep a spare pair of glasses in a well-marked place known to wife, secretary, dog, and self. 'Good boy, Broncho; bring Master's spectacles.'

3. On entering a room, survey the scene quickly to detect hidden perils like footstools and low chairs, small children lying on the floor, and other tripping hazards near the ground. Incidentally, have you noticed that even normal elderly men wearing glasses usually bow slightly on entering a room. This is known as 'bifocal politeness.'

4. Look round the room stealthily to see who is there, or you may completely miss one of its inhabitants. Quite recently I talked with a man's wife for 10 minutes in his sitting-room without observing that he also was there. Just think what might have happened.

5. Before getting up to go, make another quick survey in case someone has placed a scotch and soda on a table below your level of vision. This is more likely to occur in America than in Scotland.

6. When walking along a hospital corridor and you meet someone you know, turn your head rapidly from right to left, to make sure that he is not accompanied. In opposition to the intoxicated you are apt to see one person where there are really two. 'M. is getting so upstage nowadays; I was going along the corridor with Green when he came up and shook hands with Green and ignored me completely. He might at least have smiled.'

7. In traffic always look several times to left and right before crossing. In America and the United Kingdom you use the pedestrian crossings, but in most European countries they are better avoided, for reasons of safety. In the city where I live the 'passages de secours' are ill-placed, ill-marked, and universally ignored by drivers.

8. Don't try to read too long at one time. A half-hour spell, followed by a rest of 10 minutes, is generally enough. The rest period must not be filled in with other eye-straining activities, like television or mending your socks. It should be mental as well as an ophthalmic relaxation, a folding of the hands.

9. Avoid occupations that require a great deal of bending, such as certain forms of gardening, automobile repairs and lifting heavy articles. After all, what is a wife for?

10. I have personally found that the contemplation of rapidly moving objects gives me a sense of strain. This applies to the cinema, and to watching swiftly moving games, but not to the slower pace of the theatre. Lucky are those who are fond of music, and thinking long, long thoughts.

Chapter 18

THE SWING OF THE PENDULUM

Many centuries ago it was observed that, when a pendulum swings in one direction it is apt to return to very nearly the same point in the opposite direction. In other words, we tend to run to extremes. When I first entered preventive medicine a generation ago, one of my first jobs was to attend infant welfare centres, as they were called. Most of the clinics were held in church halls in country villages, or in elderly schools degraded to serve as village halls. They were generally dark, cold, hard-benched and uninviting. This did not matter very much to the staff, because they were filled with one gospel which they preached in and out of season: it was that infants should be fed by the clock, exactly at three (or four) hourly intervals, as recommended by the doctor. Deviation from the rule spelt disaster. Neglect of the rule meant death. Today the pendulum is at its opposite pole (or whatever you call it): the baby is fed on demand, that is, when the baby demands, however inconvenient it may be for the mother. But no; an ex-student of mine writes from an eastern territory, saying:—'We now feed the baby on demand, that is, when the mother can be bothered and has nothing else to do.' She much prefers the new system, because it imposes no duties on her. So much easier to use her breast as a comforter, when the baby becomes tiresome. What a contrast this is with the experience many years ago of a friend of mine who was a distinguished pediatrician, and his wife also, who stuck to the four hours ritual and left their infant to cry in the garden until the clock struck. Before long they received a court summons for neglect, issued by the Society for the Prevention of Cruelty to Children. Nowadays, the mother's breast can do no wrong and the baby is always right. My daughter (who has a small baby) tells me that she wakes up at night and *moos*, long before the baby is ready to demand food. This is unfortunate, but of course Nature never errs. The mother's breast is the fountain of food, affection, mental health, the prevention of delinquency, and at the same time the ever-ready faucet for the demanding infant. Pity the poor brat who has to be artificially fed; he is practically certain to be a nit-wit or a criminal. But there is worse to come. Want of mother love, possibly because the mother is dead or divorced, means that the poor babe is deprived of something absolutely vital to its physical and mental health. A bad home, we are told, is better than a good institution; and we have recently discovered that a hospital is a dreadful place because of the tensions it creates in the child, the parents, and indeed, the elderly as well. Once upon a time the hospital was a hazard to physical health on account of the danger of sepsis. It has recovered from that risk only to become a disruptive influence on the young child, to be entered with prayer and exorcism. I was a grossly deprived child myself, and I sometimes wonder what all the fuss is about; but odd delinquent strains are no doubt more obvious to others than to me. The evidence of levity on such a serious subject is enough to condemn me as abnormal. Please note that I am not advocating institutional life, but I don't think it is as dreadful as is often suggested. I have seen much human kindliness and affection in institutions, and many happy children, even at the younger ages.

Not so very long ago, the general hospital had the tidy little function of treating the sick and trying to restore them to health. Most of them, large and small alike, did this job faithfully according to their lights, and within the limits set by the medical knowledge of the times. The little units of small towns and villages were usually staffed by local general physicians who called in consultant and specialist help when they thought it was needed, or when the patient's relatives demanded it. The larger general hospitals, and more particularly those associated with medical schools, were as a rule staffed by consultants and specialists. In the days of my childhood many of these were in general practice at the same time and were consultant physicians. Gradually, as scientific medicine advanced, the specialists became more specialised and the consultants more esoteric. We then had a race of great white chiefs who made a triumphal morning round of their wards and advised their junior staff on diagnosis and treatment. Brilliant comets they were, followed by a tail of little meteors—junior housemen, medical students, austere sisters and nervous young nurses. Let us be quite fair: they were generally, in my recollection, pleasant and kind to the rather apprehensive patients. But not all. At any rate, the consultants were objects of awe and admiration.

On rare occasions a curious object was seen during this royal tour of the hospital wards: a general practitioner. Usually the great chief called him 'Tommy' or 'Billy', which showed that they had been at school or college together. We students were never taught anything about these people, and it was not brought home to us that their job was their destiny. The whole attention of the hospital, from the senior surgeon or physician to the first-year clinical student, from the medical director to the ward-maid, was concentrated on the in-patients— the sick *in bed*, and that of course is what the word *clinical* means. The outpatient department was a place in the noisome bowels of the hospital where poor patients waited for a long time on hard benches and ultimately had teeth or tonsils torn out, or an abscess evacuated, by a young surgeon surrounded by a bevy of admiring students. At stated hours, or a good deal later, a senior surgeon came down and dealt with the more serious or difficult conditions, and often combined this with a demonstration to the students. The great white chief was never seen; nor, for that matter, was a general practitioner. The outpatient department was at best a treating place, never a meeting place. Yet, more than half a century ago the great physician, Sir James Mackenzie, urged that the out-patient department was the true centre for the senior staff, because it was the only place where *early* diagnosis could be undertaken, and a study of the patient made against the background of his environment.

Still further outside the realm of our experience, as students, was the Health Officer. Once, for a few weeks, a strange person emerged from some unknown place of hibernation and delivered lectures on public health. He was regarded at best as a form of relaxation, and at worst as a bad joke; the subject he taught had apparently nothing to do with medicine, and any demonstrations he gave could be safely ignored. There was no connection between prevention and hospital care, and remarkably little association between hospital treatment and the social and working conditions to which the patient had to return after discharge. After the second world war there was a major swing of the pendulum towards the opposite extreme. It has been urged that preventive and curative medicine cannot be separated on any logical principle, and that the hospital should undertake leadership in both, as well as in the promotion of health. This claim was made by a number of the participants in the technical discussions at the World Health Assembly, held at Geneva in May, 1957. Can the claim be justified? The actual subject for discussion was 'The Role of the Hospital in the Public Health Programme.'

The right answer depends on our concept of the functions of a hospital. The first point is that the definition has been enlarged by common consent to denote a service rather than an institution, or group of institutions such as one would find in a regional scheme. Someone said that it had become an integral part of the medical and social organisation of a country, with a duty to provide comprehensive health care for its population. Its services, the statement goes on, should reach from the highest degree of teaching and research right through to the family in its home environment. Its great task would therefore be to link together all aspects of the healing art and bind with them the prevention of disease and the promotion of health. At this point many would argue that the pendulum has fairly swung off the scale. It would not be difficult to bring forward arguments to prove that the claim is exaggerated, even if we admit that the hospital service should be a health service.

Let us try to picture what are the limits of hospital service in the broad acres of public health. In the first place it obviously does not cover the environmental health services in the strict sense, including water supply and sewage disposal; nor does it make its way through the health-promoting intricacies of physical education in schools, or the organisation in the factory of an industrial health service. Health education in general and school health work in particular are outside its scope, because they are fundamentally educational services which have no conceivable connection with hospital care. On the other hand the hospital services have a vital function, previously too often misunderstood, of carrying the sick and the injured right through to the fullest possible functional health. It is no longer morally possible for the hospital to provide medical care for the sick and the injured only so long as they are occupying a hospital bed: its duty now extends to rehabilitation and indeed covers the whole range of health care from the moment of injury or sickness to the time of return to functional capacity. It does not include that part of rehabilitation which is represented by industrial retraining; this ought to be undertaken in the factory or workshop.

The principle of the major need. The rationale of this principle may be illustrated by a simple example taken from the school health service. Mary was getting on well with her school work and thinking in terms of a college education when it became clear to the ophthalmologist that her high myopia was dangerously progressive and that she would become totally blind. Her mother—an intelligent woman—asked the consultant what should be done in the meantime. He replied that she should live quietly and avoid anything that might lead to eyestrain. Would this be likely to prolong the period of useful eyesight? The specialist thought that with care there should be a delay of some two or three years before the onset of total blindness, if she were careful. 'But,' said the mother, 'Mary is a good student and is learning rapidly; if there was a break just at this moment in her learning, she would have great difficulty in ever picking up the threads again.' Said the specialist, 'That is your responsibility. I have to advise you that if Mary goes on reading now, she will inevitably sacrifice a period of sight in her twenties.' He was no doubt quite right in his own sphere, but he had not learned the principle of the major need, which would have told him that continuity of education was the major need, to store up riches of mind and memory in preparation for the darkness to come. It was beautifully expressed long ago: 'I must work the works of him that sent me, while it is day; for the night cometh when no man can work.'

The position of children suffering from other forms of physical handicap follows the same principle. The hospital service has special functions. In the case of a child partially paralysed as a result of poliomyelitis, for example, the duty of rehabilitation begins at once and goes on without a break until the fullest possible functional restoration has been achieved. First, there is the physical handicap: the main risks are regression from want of exercise aimed at maintaining a balanced progress in the use of *all* the limbs. The out-patient services have also a duty to guard against disuse atrophy from outgrown apparatus or from neglect in use. A further function cannot be ignored, although it may be employed indirectly through school or industry: that is, to make sure that the patient is not placed in an awkward position in school or factory or in such a posture as to promote deformity or contracture. The outpatient department must now assume this elementary duty of after-care. Even this is not enough: the crippled child has to be restored to normal psychological function. Many of them suffer from that 'left behind' feeling, which leads to either aggressive tendencies or to undue timidity—but always to a sense of inferiority. The follow-up service has to be on its guard against excessive 'protection' by the parents, as this inevitably leads to undue concentration on the disability. Self-pity may be aroused by over-sympathy, and want of self-help by an excessive effort to keep up with normal children. The most serious illustration of this principle, however, is the risk of making a double handicap by failure to secure continuous and progressive education. The creation of a child crippled by disease or accident is a tragedy of life; but failure to educate him is the tragedy of a living death. There are splints to support a weak limb, but none for a disused mind. Some years ago we made a survey of the educational provision for children in a group of our larger hospitals providing *general* care for the sick. We found a considerable number of children who had been in-patients for periods up to eighteen months without having received any education worth the name. If this can happen to in-patients, what about the children receiving general out-patient care, but not yet ready for school? Rehabilitation includes a duty to the mind as well as to the body.

Chapter 19

. AMERICAN PILGRIMAGE IN WARTIME

PRELUDE IN LISBON, 1941

We live from hand to mouth in one of the few international oases of the world. Lisbon is a town of colour and light to the stranger who has just escaped from the blackness of a British city. His first impulse is to sit up half the night by an open window revelling in the gay advertisement signs, the brilliant street lamps, and the swift movement of traffic. Then he lies in bed reading, with curtains undrawn and all his lights burning; and at last, after tossing restlessly through the early hours of the morning, he begins to wish that the citizens of Lisbon were less devoted to the sound of motor-horns.

There are three worlds in Lisbon today. The first consists of the great ones of the earth—Ambassadors, their secretaries, and their typists. We call them 'The Grand Priorities', because they come and go as they please, spurning the common earth with their majestic pinions. We the second world, are the flotsam and jetsam of the high seas, all trying to find an insignificant corner in some outward-bound plane or ship. We arrived, it may be, from Britain some weeks ago, full of the importance of our business mission to the United States, loaded with visas, and girded with petty priorities. Or we have been working with the Red Cross in Timbuctoo, and they do not want us any more. Perhaps we had vineyards in Madeira or Oporto and used to carry on a noble business with Britain, and now want to go home and help in a more personal way.

On the other hand, we may be British wives of American citizens, or just pleasant American women who have somehow strayed into the unlovely garden of Europe. At any rate, we are all here united by two consuming passions—first, hatred of the 'Grand Priorities', whose passage means that our reservation is once again postponed; and, secondly, the desire to get away somehow.

Omnes eodem cogimur, omnium
Versatur urna serius ocius
Sors exitura. . .

By which Horace probably meant—'We're all in the same show;
maybe sooner, maybe later, we'll throw a double-six and get
out'.

Conversation at dinner always returns to the same topic:
'I wonder if the Clipper came in yesterday' or 'Do you know
of any Consuls who are crossing this week'? Apart from this
obsession, international table-talk is generally interesting. One
night my knowledge of German was just sufficient to translate—
'S-sh! Do not talk so loud; there are English swine on your
right'. Immediately the clear voice of the girl with the flaxen
hair cut across the table—'Well, if it's economic planning you
mean, and not a spiritual reconstruction, I guess you've gotten
the wrong . . .' and this, too, trails away, or is lost in the
delicious honeydew melon that sucks about my ears.

The third world is Lisbon, the national city of the Portuguese.
This has a more abiding interest, because one feels that the
everyday human things go on, undismayed by the tempests
overhead. Street-cars grind up impossible hills and automobiles
swing round perilous corners with a gay abandon, careless of
untended human sheep like me. The staunch, straight-backed
women come up from market with loaded baskets on their
heads, making practical use of the ridiculous woollen things
which our girls twist round their hair. The men ply their
various trades at open shop-fronts, and the wiry, mischievous
brats try to sell week-old newspapers to innocent exiles.

If you want to visit slums in Lisbon and see how the people
really live, you will be well advised to take with you a dimpled,
sedate, America-trained public health nurse who knows her
job. Otherwise you will get into trouble in the Rua Silva o
Albuquerque and require a generous application of the Pos de
Keating so much advertised on the street-cars.

One of my first visits was to the combined house and workshop of a coffin-maker, where the eternal and the temporal
resting-place stood cheek by jowl. The tiny bedrooms had only
internal ventilation to a passage, but they were clean and fresh.
In the next house a most ingenious method had been devised
to meet the needs of a steadily increasing family. The house

was old, with high rooms, so a rough 'upper deck' had been inserted between floor and ceiling. This little room, reached by a ladder, had, of course, no external ventilation, and borrowed its light from the main window. Its total area of five feet by eight managed to hold a double bed for the three girls, but that was all.

Another woman lived in an old stable, where she kept her numerous progeny in the mangers and used the main building as kitchen and sitting-room. Her little charcoal stove was busy with the latest baby's milk.

In many of the poorer houses, like the cottages of Old England, the height from floor to ceiling is less than six feet. Yet, in spite of obvious poverty and wretched clothing for beds and bodies, there was an agreeable absence of smell. The sun is a great purifier, and he finds no difficulty in reaching the deep courts and alleys on these precipitous hillsides. Even the poorest are fond of washing clothes and hanging the rags on gay lines to catch the sunlight. But, on the whole, the standard of living is low, and the small number of calories on which the children live would shock our nutrition experts.

The lithe, bright-eyed children are thin, but they show little sign of rickets or gross malnutrition. I examined more or less superficially just under a thousand children and was able to pick out only a few deformed bones and a mere handful of pot-bellied, boss-headed infants. Fruit and sunlight are cheap and plentiful.

On the other hand, disease and death rates are high, especially among infants. In Britain an enormous expenditure of effort on health has brought down our infant mortality rates from 150 per 1,000 a generation ago to about 60 today. Holland and New Zealand have done far better. Lisbon is still wrestling with a rate which fluctuates around 150, at least two-thirds of which is due to preventable causes. The health service is in a state of transition between environmental and personal hygiene, and much remains to be done before a complete scheme is established.

One of the most interesting experiments in health has been the establishment in Lisbon through the generosity of the Rockefeller Foundation, of a 'demonstration' Health Centre, covering a working population of about 14,000 (out of a total

of over 700,000). Within this selected area health education
and a system of home visitation by trained nurses has been
going on for some years. The results are promising—a reduction
of 40 per cent in the infant death rate and a striking improvement in co-operation among the people. This pioneer work
points the way to a general extension of the personal health
services.

Another day of strenuous exploring is over—this time in the
deeper valleys of poverty. A hot bath relieves me of unwelcome
visitors, and dinner brings the international news—a long tale
of priorities and deferred hopes. But my withers are unwrung:
tomorrow I am going 'up country' to Torres Vedras and the
north to see remote villages and simple folk. Au revoir, Airway
offices. Your tact, patience and courtesy are beyond praise, but
I am sure you hate the sight of my face. I will lift mine eyes to
the hills. Till Monday, then, adieu.

FALTERING FIRST STEPS

The first approach to a place often colours the whole of
one's memories. The visitor to Inverness in Scotland, for
example, who arrives from East or South, can never forget the
sordid coalyard entrance which nearly ruins the beauty of the
Northern capital. The best gateway to the United States from
the East is through The Narrows in a ship, for the first vision of
the great cluster of buildings on Manhattan is one of the most
imposing things ever created by man. From the air these
splendid palaces are dwarfed against the immense background
of level continent. Although New York is a cosmopolitan city,
it represents much that is characteristic of America—many
nationalities, but one nation; and a jungle of structures of all
manner of height and design, making one city. Some time ago
a friend took me to an Italian restaurant on 21st Street and
proceeded to air his gift of tongues to the waiter. The latter
bore this patiently for two courses and then said with quiet
dignity: 'Sir, I would have you know that I am an American'.
That is the first lesson.

The second lesson begins with the growing knowledge that a
visit to the Eastern Seaboard provides only a casual and very
imperfect view of the United States, much in the same way as
a dash from Dover to London and back would count for

familiarity with the British Isles. Far too few Britons pay their respects to the great cities of the Middle West, where there is the most urgent need for mutual understanding. Chicago is perhaps the most American of all the cities and is certainly one of the most hospitable. Its isolation, so far as it now exists, reflects our lack of enterprise rather than any failure on their part. The great industrial area ought to be seen and appreciated. But we must return to the East and spend some time in Washington—the unfinished symphony. This will be the ideal National Capital, if its population can be kept within bounds. Our own great planning difficulty in Britain after the war will be to prevent the sprawl of cities by building new towns complete in themselves. Wartime overcrowding of capitals can't be helped, but we must try to put a curb on extension and not allow them to overflow like broken sewers. The beauty and grace of Washington makes one wish that we would select York rather than London as our National Capital, leaving New York and London as the great cosmopolitan centres—lovable but incorrigible.

The West should be approached by air. You leave the friendly shelter of Chicago and move with unhurrying speed across seemingly endless plains, until a halt at Cheyenne gives a first glimpse of the Rocky Mountains. The next stop is in Utah and the great pewter-coloured lake still gleams faintly in the gathering dusk; after that only the frequent bumps tell you that you are crossing ridge after ridge of the Sierra Nevada. Suddenly there are a million lights around and beneath, matching the frosty stars above. You have entered a new country, where the thoughts of the people are turned towards the Pacific; where China and Japan are far more real than Britain and Germany. Meanwhile the cheerful little stewardess is busy explaining that the long chain of lights is the Bay Bridge, crossing from Oakland to San Francisco; the Golden Gate and the dim ocean are half-imagined beyond. They played me a trick in San Francisco by taking me to a Chinese Restaurant and placing only chop-sticks beside my plate. But some years ago Dr. Jean Chiang (I wonder where she is now?) stayed with us in England and taught us all to use these strange weapons. So I emerged triumphant from the ordeal.

The next journey carried me down the whole length of the

Mississippi from Minneapolis to New Orleans, there to find another people within the Union, with strong French tradition and even speech. Louisiana, with an old, romantic world behind it, stands out in sharp contrast with its young neighbour, Texas, where new cities spring up in a night. There is nothing depressing about these great rolling plains: everything speaks of the vigour of youth, and air travel has brought all its vast distances within the little measure of a day's jaunt.

The South has a flavour of its own, and an Englishman feels very much at home there, because of the strong ties of affection between its people and the home country. The Scot is always a welcome visitor in the Carolinas where many of his ancestors penetrated the shadowed rivers, but on the whole one is reminded more of life in the English County, with its slow pace, its love of outdoor sport and its gentleness. There is no need to convert the Southerner to the British point of view; he has it already in advance. 'We are all Anglo-Saxons here' is a common form of welcome.

I take New England for granted as a place to be visited, and Canada is only a mashie shot away; but I am sure that the most important duty and privilege for men and women of goodwill who visit the United States at this time is to go to the Middle West, the West, and the South, to strengthen the friendship which is growing fast between these 'peoples' and ourselves.

THE EVE OF WAR

THANKSGIVING DAY, 1941*

I have eaten too much turkey and plum pudding, but there is a warm feeling in my heart also. Detroit, with its mighty industries hushed, wears an air of unusual solemnity, broken only by the C.I.O. Conference, which bulges out the very walls of my hotel. This morning I was awakened by a peal of ordnance, shot off apparently in honour of a procession of 'Christmas' delights for children. This is quite appropriate, for the day is dedicated to the family—and for me it bears the memory of a cheerful homely dinner and an atmosphere of gracious piety that belongs to an older world.

On reaching the Middle West I have entered a new America.

* Written a few days before Japan plunged the United States into the war.

The outlook on war has changed significantly, especially n Illinois and Minnesota, with increasing distance from the ocean. In this strange land I can now look back with some sense of perspective on the views expressed by those who live near the shores of the Atlantic. These views are held emphatically, even passionately. On the eastern seaboard the man in the street— represented in cosmopolitan New York by Thomas, Ricardo, and Heinrich—is rapidly losing his patience. These loyal and devoted citizens of the United States of America admit readily enough that their more backward countrymen had to be educated before they could appreciate the meaning of total war, and realise the danger in which they stood.

But education should lead to graduation. 'This programme', said my taxidriver, waving his arms furiously as we dashed across the corner of 57th and 5th Avenue, 'this programme should have been finished in twelve months. There's no sense in schooling us when we've learned our lesson. We are all ahead of the President now'.

This expresses an opinion widely held among all classes of people in the East that it was good statesmanship to prepare the ground for a season; astute policy, perhaps, to sow vast acres in differing soil and climate; but bad husbandry, now that the harvest is plentiful, to hold back the reapers, for some of the crops will never ripen and others will fall before the first winter storms of disunity.

The British onlooker is less downright. He retains his faith in the present Administration and approves its wise caution. Yet some of his arguments, derived mainly from the British press, are brushed impatiently aside by American friends.

Not long ago, I was studying the Gettysburg battlefield with a student of history, who referred to Lincoln's uncanny intuition in selecting the right moment for action. The glory of the autumn woods around us made war seem very far away, and the reverently tended memorials to both sides in the Civil War spoke eloquently of union after strife. My fellow-student, realising that his words implied criticism of the present Government, pulled himself back with a painful wrench to the situation of the moment, and said, a little sententiously—'There is a tide in the affairs of men—and our President has missed the flood'.

'But, surely', I demurred, 'there is a strong case for caution. Lincoln himself was assailed again and again for failure to act in times of crisis. Yet his stature grows with every passing year. If you rush into open war today you will raise an instant howl for defence of your own coasts. Those who cling to isolation, and many more also, will clamour against sending munitions abroad until America is armed to the teeth. You will be playing into the hands of the enemy within your gates'.

'No, no', he replied, 'you don't understand the American. What we need more than anything else is the stimulus of war against us. One touch of that sharp goad will bring unity of effort, and we should soon be producing enough for ourselves, and far more for you at the same time. Until we are fully into the war we can't put forth our strength. At the moment we are just playing at what you call a " 'keep fit campaign' ".

I tried again—'Yes, but can it not be said that your nation is at war already? Your Navy ranges over the seas and suffers loss with ours: its convoy ships are ready to take every risk'.

'This is mere casuistry', he answered, 'although it goes down with our people and many of yours. Sticky half-truths like that are candy to childish consciences. Suck and sleep'.

I was silent, because I had no ready answer; but later in the day, as we picked our steps in the fading light along the Appalachian Trail, doubts began to crowd upon me. A good many of our American friends, I thought, find it difficult to dissociate domestic and foreign policy. In their unconscious minds they feel that they cannot approve the one and condemn the other without setting up an unpleasant conflict. You may love a friend and swallow his faults whole without indigestion, but a President is another matter.

Possibly a man might be found to satisfy both domestic and foreign policies. An opinion like this is seldom expressed, because it is not brought into the conscious mind. Many of the doubters read the lesson of history well enough to be aware that their own vision may be restricted. The one man who is in a position to see things steadily and see things whole is the President, and there are no doubt many reasons why he should stay his hand.

It is sometimes assumed that he is waiting only until public opinion is moulded, but there are other and perhaps stronger motives in the strategy of war. My last tired thought, as we passed out of the darkened forest into the warm light of a mountain inn, was as disconnected as my steps: Well, after all, in a democracy those who shout loudest are generally in a minority; under dictatorship the same thing may occur. At a critical period of the Civil War the editor of 'The Spectator' said—'The American Republic is not in times of excitement governed by its talking class'.

We are often told that the Americans are a sentimental people—and so they are. That is one reason why we Scots feel so much at home in their company. This morning I was on my way down the marble steps after my third visit to the Lincoln Memorial at Washington. An American sailor who was walking slowly by my side was suddenly hailed by a friend: 'Hello boy, what you doin' here?' My companion put on a facetious air and drawled 'I was jist up to look if th' ole man was still there; must be darn' tired sittin' on that marble chair'. I looked round and noticed that the speaker's eyes were as wet as mine.

This little incident gave me a clue to something that puzzled me about American sentiment. We in Britain are inclined to look too lightly upon what is really a deep internal conflict, if we imagine that the issue of the moment lies simply between peace and war, delay and action. The memory of Abraham Lincoln is enshrined in the hearts of his people because he gave their diffuse sentiment a dynamic force and purpose; and the great memorial at Washington is profoundly moving to all who love America, not only on account of the beauty of its design, but also because it makes us 'feel the inly touch' of democratic ideals.

The citizen of the United States is anxious and troubled today; he is waiting for a leader to restate his faith in plain words and give him a clear call to action. The time is at hand.

MANY VOICES, 1942

On returning from flying visits to the half-dozen nations which constitute the United States of America I am disturbed to find that many people at home regard 'American opinion' as something which is, or ought to be, homogeneous. This is equivalent to including in 'British opinion' the views of the inhabitants of the United Kingdom, Eire, Australia, Canada, and South Africa.

Historians point out that the sentiment which draws separate peoples towards federation depends upon two feelings which are to some extent inconsistent—a desire for unity and a determination on the part of each group to maintain its independence. An important element in federation is that the members of the various groups feel a stronger allegiance to their own traditions and ways of life than to the central government, but are nevertheless willing to be welded together for certain common purposes.

There are forty-eight States in the Union, but sentiment and tradition cover wider and less well defined areas than those somewhat artificial State boundaries. Some of the groupings stand out clearly as though legally recognized lines had been drawn around them. Others, like our Highlands and our border areas, have a character of their own and draw their strength from traditional loyalties.

So it is with New England, the South, the Deep South, and the South-West. The Industrial North-East, the Middle West, and the West Coast are perhaps more determined by geographical position than by ties of sentiment; but their right to a point of view is none the less real.

All this goes to suggest that there is no such thing as American opinion, and that the visitor who confines his attentions to New York and Washington can know little of the American people, even if he listens from afar to isolationist murmurings out of the Middle West.

He is apt to forget that Chicago is 800 miles from the Atlantic and nearly twice that distance from the Pacific Ocean. The good and kindly people in the Middle West are in fact isolated, and it is perfectly natural that they should feel remote from war in Europe and Asia and remain more or less indifferent to Britain's struggle. That will be the position until we tell them about *our* work and constantly restate our ideals. Even that is not enough: We must tell them how much we appreciate their help, and how much they can do to lighten our task.

Some years ago a friend of mine joined the ranks of the blood donors. No doubt he felt a vague satisfaction in contributing his quota to the 'pool', but his imagination was fired when a

letter came to tell him that his blood had been given to a
seriously injured child, and that the patient had made a good
recovery. This personal touch is no longer possible either in
blood-giving or in blood letting, but the spirit of the thing lives
on.

The British Library of Information in New York strains all
its resources to give a fair deal to the Middle West, but it needs
more support from the British authorities and the press; less
yelping and petty criticism, and more positive news about our
war work, our achievements, and our ideals.

The picture of a Britain that is always 'taking it', facing
misfortune, understating its sentiments, and criticising its
Government is not a stimulating offering to the New World.
The Americans are friendly and eagerly responsive to gestures
of confidence and of affection.

In New England and in the warm South they can stand a
good deal of coldness on our part without complaint, but
farther West they are more sensitive. Their warm-heartedness
is sometimes chilled by our apparent failure to make allowance
for the difficulties peculiar to the Middle Western States, and
anti-British feeling is easily aroused by criticism of shortcomings
in these great arsenals of democracy.

Let us try to promote a better understanding with the Middle
West and make them feel a sense of real co-operation and
helpfulness. As the war goes on, it should not be possible to say
of any group or section of the two great nations that,

> They fed not on the advancing hours . . .
> Then each applied to each that fatal knife.
> Deep-questioning, that probes to endless dole.

My task in the United States was to advise on certain aspects
of civil defence. My advice was of little value until I studied the
American background and understood what a vast difference
there had to be in practice between the two countries. Knowledge of this kind cannot be acquired in a few weeks, nor is it
possible to give intelligent guidance without examining at first
hand the widely diverging problems of the Atlantic and the
Pacific Coasts, the Mexican Gulf, and the Mid-Western States.

My final suggestion would be that we should send more men
and women to the United States—people with first-hand
experience of present-day Britain and with detailed knowledge

T

of their own spheres of work, educational, social, medical, and so on. We should send them farther afield and for periods of not less than six months. These people should learn before they begin to teach. They do not need to know anything about propaganda or politics, but they should know how to make friends and to talk simply about the ordinary people of Britain, their everyday life and work, and their efforts to create good out of evil.

I have no doubt that the grown-ups who are experts in diplomacy or steel, or food-purchasing are invaluable in Washington—but don't send them to Texas. Look gently at Houston, which a few decades ago was a wilderness and is now a thriving, beautiful city of 600,000 inhabitants. How gloriously young it is! Don't send old stiffs there, but people who are fresh and young, with romance and sentiment in their hearts. The Middle West also is young. There is little room for the hard-boiled. If you want anybody for California, Oregon or Washington State, send me.

THE PACIFIC COAST

To leave New York in the evening and come to rest on the Pacific Coast in time for lunch the following day is a light undertaking. It is a heavier matter if, by some rare chance of weather, you are decanted at four in the morning on a prairie at a temperature of 20 degrees below zero; but the final translation to the sunshine of the West is all the richer for that experience. Now I understand why people who come here from the Middle West never go back again. I have no intention of returning either. The rest of my life will be spent in eating the oranges that fall in my lap and watching the idle ocean.

The citizens of the Western seaboard are just as conscious of war as their fellows in the East, and perhaps more keenly alive to the need for civil defence. The first blow struck nearer home and the remoter effects of that treachery are still being treated as a septic wound.

But it is a different war here: the raucous voice of Hitler has a long way to travel and only a faint confused echo succeeds in crossing the prairies and the rugged mountains of Nevada. The Japanese are real enough, however, and the eternal grin takes on a peculiarly sinister quality at this distance.

This increases the sense of urgency in planning, but the civil authorities find difficulty in passing from the stage of conference to their action stations. This trouble is partly local and partly due to the immense distance from the Federal capital.

There is much to be said for giving a greater measure of autonomy to the West in war-time even to the extent of setting up a federal office with wide executive authority. At the same time too much devolution is to be deprecated: the seven or eight States of the far West should hang together as one unit of government.

In Britain we had the same confusion during the early days of the war, and much good paper was wasted before we realised that civilian defence plans cannot be made effective without central direction and control, and that at the same time the country ought to be split up into sizable regions to hold the smaller areas together.

It is harder for the United States to devise such a scheme, because it has three levels of control: the Federal Government, the 48 States, and the local authorities who are as the sands in number. Under peace-time conditions the latter are like a couple of small Scottish burghs who happen to have boundaries in common. A good defence programme cannot tolerate local jealousies; its basis is mutual aid.

One lesson which has not yet been fully learnt in the United States is the immense value to public morale of civilian, as a supplement to military, defence. There is an unfortunate tendency in some quarters to fold the hands and say—'Well, if the civil authority cannot do this the Army will step in and carry out the task, declaring martial law if necessary'.

Now, the supreme success of civilian defence in Britain has been the result of two main factors: that the people have learned to put their trust in their own right arm to meet the menace from the sky, and they have not been found wanting.

The second factor is that women have been enabled to stand by their menfolk in equality of sacrifice and courage. These contributions to the strength of Great Britain have been of inestimable value, and have brought light to all the days of darkness. The Army is a weapon of offence; the people themselves, men and women alike, are the rock of our defence.

Sitting here in the sunshine, I have been wondering how technical officers from Great Britain can render their best services to America. My sands are running out, and I am now in a position to review experience and reach some pretty definite conclusions.

The first and most important point is that it is not our business to instruct our American colleagues what to do. Our duty is to watch their activities and illuminate them by illustrations of fact from British experience. Secondly, we must be thoroughly versed in the details of our subject.

The next rule of conduct is to tell the truth, and to tell it as simply as possible. The time for propaganda is long past, and the time for circumlocution never existed in the United States.

And, lastly, the British visitor must resist the temptation to become 'Sir Oracle'. Many men and women, well informed on their own subjects, have allowed themselves to be drawn into a vortex of publicity. Before long their 'gracious messages from the throne' cover the whole range of politics, economics, and social welfare. The British 'expert' should be content with the workshop and not aspire to the stage; it is there that he is most useful and least in the way.

'Tell us before you go how you like the Americans.' I can only answer by quoting a little verse which I wrote to one representative American on St. Valentine's Day in New York:—

> I cannot tell a finished story;
> My days are fragments—here a dream
> And there an arch through which the glory
> Of Golden Gate and golden sunset gleam.

> I cannot equal your deserving,
> Nor would you ask a recompense
> Save friendship, loyalty unswerving
> To common faith. Against this pestilence

> Of war our nations have united
> Their strength to bring deliverance
> From fear. When wrongs have been requited,
> Will they resume their old inheritance

Unchanging? This fantastic city,
  Sky-searching, sheds ten million lights
Into the dusk; the Spirit of Pity,
  Brooding at first from the eternal heights,

Sees only symbols, tragic, brittle,
  Of feeble vision; and the brave
Majestic buildings as a little
  Embossed memorial on a country grave.

But she descends, for deeper knowing;
  And draws aside the prison bars,
Till you and I can see the glowing,
  Serene Horizon, and above—the stars.

Printed by
George Outram & Co. Ltd.,
36 Tay Street, Perth.